HISTOPATHOLOGY - AN UPDATE

Edited by **Supriya Srivastava**

Histopathology - An Update
http://dx.doi.org/10.5772/intechopen.69367
Edited by Supriya Srivastava

Contributors

Arbab Sikandar, Ilze Strumfa, Ilze Fridrihsone, Andrejs Vanags, Dainis Balodis, Arnis Abolins, Boriss Strumfs, Arvids Jakovlevs, Janis Gardovskis, Kinan Drak Alsibai, Didier Meseure, Imad Elimairi, Hind Alkatan, Tariq Al-Zahem, José Carlos Tavares Carvalho, Gisele Custódio De Souza, Irlon Maciel Ferreira, Helison De Oliveira Carvalho, Igor Victor Ferreira Dos Santos, Giovanna Rocha Santana, Jonatas Lobato Duarte, Caio Pinho Fernandes, Hady Keita, José Luis Balderas-Lopez, Andrés Navarrete Castro

First published in London, United Kingdom, 2018 by IntechOpen
IntechOpen is the global imprint of INTECHOPEN LIMITED, registered in England and Wales, registration number: 11086078, The Shard, 25th floor, 32 London Bridge Street
London, SE19SG – United Kingdom
Printed in Croatia

British Library Cataloguing-in-Publication Data
A catalogue record for this book is available from the British Library

Additional hard copies can be obtained from orders@intechopen.com

Histopathology - An Update, Edited by Supriya Srivastava
p. cm.
Print ISBN 978-1-78923-686-6
Online ISBN 978-1-78923-687-3

For EU product safety concerns:
IN TECH d.o.o., Prolaz Marije Krucifikse Kozulić 3, 51000 Rijeka, Croatia,
info@intechopen.com or visit our website at intechopen.com.

Meet the editor

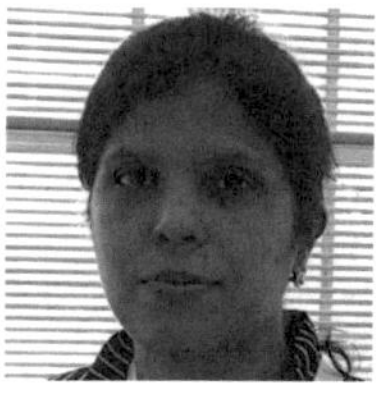

Dr Supriya Srivastava (MBBS, MD Pathology) is a Research Fellow in Department of Medicine, YLLSOM, National University of Singapore. Her areas of interest include, gastrointestinal tract tumors and identifying biomarkers in early diagnosis of GIT tumors. She has an expertise in immunohistochemistry; immunofluorescence, FISH and laser capture microdissection. She published around 30 papers as first author and co-author in per-reviewed international journals.

Contents

Preface

Science is constantly evolving and every day there are new discoveries and breakthroughs. In the clinical field, histopathology plays a major role in patient outcomes. Histopathology is an age-old technique used to study the anatomy of normal and diseased tissues. Histopathology was, in the past and still continues to be the gold standard for diagnosis. In recent times, to aid the pathologists, there have been innumerable advances in pathology. Mostly these advances are in the field of discoveries of molecular biomarkers. These biomarkers can help the pathologists in diagnosing a difficult lesion or also in differentiating a lesion with its closest differential diagnosis. Therefore it is imperative that the pathologists are abreast of the latest knowledge in this field. To help the pathologists, clinicians, researchers and residents, the esteemed panel of authors are pleased to publish this book, which is an update in the field of histopathology.

The chapters though limited, yet they bring the latest update in that particular field. The content of this book ranges from general pathology to organ specific histopathology. This book highlights advances in histology and histopathology that could help the pathologists in reaching a diagnosis in a better away. Each chapter is well illustrated with colored figures and tables and charts are provided to aid in the better understanding of the content of the chapters. Each chapter has been reviewed and tailored to the needs of the readers.

I appreciate and am deeply thankful to the authors for their hard work in publishing this book. I also feel obliged to thank the IntechOpen publishers for making me a part of this book. In addition, I would like to thank Mr. Slobodan Momcilovic and the technical staff who helped me whenever I reached out to them. Lastly, I would like to express my gratitude to my family for supporting me through this journey.

Dr. Supriya Srivastava
Yong Loo Lin School of Medicine
National University of Singapore
Singapore

Section 1

General Pathology

Chapter 1

Histopathology: An Old Yet Important Technique in Modern Science

Arbab Sikandar

Additional information is available at the end of the chapter

http://dx.doi.org/10.5772/intechopen.76908

Abstract

Histopathology is a scientific study of disease at the tissue and cellular levels. Despite an old practice, the histopathology reserved one of the substantial sections of disease studies, both and medical and veterinary field in the modern scientific era. During the current molecular age, some improvements have been made in this practice. The early modification in histopathology is the introduction of immunohistochemistry, which playing an incredible role in tumor diagnosis. The new developments, including digital pathology, multiplex immunohistochemistry, immunofluorescence, brain mapping, neuroimaging studies and artificial neuronal networking are emphasizing novel technologies and almost changed the previous ordinary diagnostic methods. The existing molecular pathobiology, was evolved mainly from biopsy and autopsy. Currently, the revolutions in molecular biology and in the technology of gene array have developed. The telepathology helping the society and deals with histopathological pictures. It is not far, when molecular techniques would be applied to the lesions prior to its paraffinizations, and the histopathological experts would previously recognize what to study in the sections. The productive move from a visual morphological explanation to obscure molecular science, may be delay, but ultimately be there. This chapter tries to express few of such characteristics of the histopathological practice which assured to be the fast progressing portion of the modern science.

Keywords: histopathology, developing countries, diagnosis

1. Introduction

Histopathology is being exercised in most parts of the world and is still in the developmental phase in various developing countries. This branch contributes a significant portion in the cutting edge effective diagnosis in pathology through highlighting the unique microarchitecutral and morphological results. For long, the histopathologists studied their pathological diagnostic reports exclusively on the tissue growth patterns and cell morphology with usual heamatoxylin and eosin (H&E) and few (if any) special stained slides. Today's developed technology makes the computerized histomorphometric diagnosis and prognosis possible, and now the results are more scientific and reproducible. The gene array measures thousands of gene expression, facilitating the researcher for pursuing new and rapid markers for disease diagnosis. By this way a molecular diagnosis of the pathological lesions would derived prior to the preparation of paraffinized sections. The micro array analysis of DNA and proteomics make likely to figure a comprehensive gene expression belongs to tissue neoplasia and helps in diagnosis, susceptibility and prognosis. Such tests are being done in conjunction with preceding histopathology for better results. Artificial neuronal networking is introduced by a surgical pathologist in whom an artificial neuron is working like physiologically normal one by passing information. The telepathology is dealing with obtaining, spreading, and broadcasting of histopathological pictures through the telecommunication networks viz. internet and satellite. This practice will make the study of whole-slide easy and will let the prompt distributions of the images for early diagnosis and detail disease process. Now most of the short-commings are being overcomed and the imminent archetype of histopathology is hypothesized to be digital in the near future. By this means the histopathologists will confirm diagnosis via virtual images analysis on computers instead of as usual morphometry and the digitized tissue could categorize into various histological grading for quantitative analysis, which results in provision of rapid and improved prospects for diagnosis and treatment of tumorous tissues. In the current thrilling time of pathology, we are challenged with the novel boundary of cutting-edge science and technology, which progress and speed up the diagnostic histopathological technique. But still it is not less than a challenge for achieving such procedures successfully so as to route all the information enclosed.

2. History

The histopathology refers to the examination of prepared tissue under microscopic and the practice is however in the development phase in most of the developing countries [1]. It has been found that most of the important lesions which are easy to get during biopsy are still not biopsied in those countries and if so, then most of the important surgically isolated tissues are not being processed accurately for histopathology. Most of the existing gaps that need to be filled is the lack of availability of important good quality chemicals, reagents and instruments viz. unavailability of Microtomes for fine sectioning and electron microscopes for tissue study etc., and unavailability of various very common tests including, immunohistochemistry. Various teaching and research institutes are lacking these facilities and are focusing on H&E only [2]. The concept of staining a tissue is for clear visualization of its microstructure. Most commonly used eosin is an acidic coloring chemical that stains basic structures having negatively charge i.e. the cytoplasm. The other companion color is the hematoxylin which is basic in nature and is imparting the color to the acidic portion of the cell i.e. nucleus [3]. Special staining of the tissue is also out of use, but, if available, then its results will not be appropriate. Only few private sectors are claiming that they are producing the slides of a good quality, but the methods are still needed to be standardized. If in case any slide is made up as per routine use of advanced countries, there is a bridge of availability of technically trained persons who can read the slides exactly. State of the art facility of equipment's needed to available along with skilled personals that can get the specimens, processed, stained and could read the lesions. The tumor pathology practice is increasing with the time [4] and the histopathology practice is also needs to be rectified as this is a tool of diagnosing the tumor rapidly and is reliable [5]. The developing countries need to accurate the practice of histopathology with the intention that they could help the civilians in diagnosing the existing regional disease conditions. So that the pictures of good results could be cited in international literature. The histopathology is skinning new grace in finding cause and pathogenesis of diseases [5]. A lot of developing countries faced funding's, trained technicians, equipment's and materials problems [6]. One of the emerging trends in the current scientific era is invention of digital histopathology [7], which is considered as a break-through and celebrity in finding and studying numerous varieties of cancers. The current chapter highlighting the use and application of histopathological old techniques and also highlighting the simultaneous use of old and emerging new techniques in the field of histopathology and also debated about its future recommendations.

3. Position of histopathology in the modern science

Disease is developed from the molecular level followed by cellular and tissue level [8]. It is utmost necessary to grab any disease in the stage when it creates changes in the tissues [9]. In histopathology we study scientifically the changes in the affected tissues under the microscope. Though this is an ancient procedure, and still being adopted in medical sciences [10]. This section of pathology enjoying a considerable portion of detail study of most of the humans as well as animal ailments. This outlet of scientific study reserved a substantial position in the modern techniques in effective disease diagnosis. In histopathology the micro-architectural detail of tissue is being highlighted. For this the tissues are being stained with various categories of stains. Although this practice is a time consuming process, however, some improvements have been made in such protocol during the modern era. The new developments in the current novel technologies improved the earlier conventional disease diagnostic procedures, making enabled such practice in a rapid way [11]. The manual protocol is replaced with the automated machines. In recent times the histological image of life sciences is processed in medical sciences, same to that of the engineer [12]. Tremendous improvements have been made in such medical image processing technology. Due to the improvement of the information technology, the tissue imaging technique is the most acceptable, efficient and reliable mean to detect the cancer and other diseases.

4. Improvements in histopathology

The histopathology is being practiced sidewise to the molecular techniques in the technologically developed world, and the less developed countries are still competing to standardize such technique. The experts in histopathology used the prepared slides entirely on growth patterns, infiltrated cells and tissue morphology with ordinary staining protocol [5]. The H&E staining are widely being used in histopathology and currently, various specific stains are being established [12]. The aim of these stains is to identify the specific affected tissues after imparting it with different dye. Several special stains have been developed and are being practiced successfully in renowned established laboratories. The special stained make the slides easy in differentiation and identification, which are then subjected into rapid computerized histomorphometric diagnosis.

5. Position of histopathology in the modern diagnostics

The major ailment around the world is the cancer and is considered as a chronic disease of the age [13]. Numerous death rates owing to cancer have been reported in human and animal population, and its rate is increasing astonishingly with time. The foremost change and upgradation in histopathology is through the use of immunohistochemical methods [11], which playing an incredible role in tumor diagnosis. The applicable prognosis and early diagnosis of biopsy specimens is possible, and the scientific results obtained are now more reproducible. Other than disease diagnosis, most of the tissues are being developed in the laboratories through culture methods [14]. The tissue culture labs are the leading player of the tissues being cultured. These labs recently claimed the culturing and the introduction of the artificial neuronal networking, in whom an artificial neuron is working like physiologically normal one by passing signals and effective information [15].

The existing molecular pathobiology was evolved mainly from biopsy and autopsy [8]. Currently, the revolutions in molecular biology and in the technology of gene array have developed which measures thousands of genes expression, facilitating the researcher for pursuing new and rapid markers for disease diagnosis [14]. By this way a molecular diagnosis of the pathological lesions would derived prior to the preparation of paraffinized sections. The micro array analysis of DNA and proteomics make likely to figure a comprehensive gene expression belongs to tissue neoplasia and helps in diagnosis, susceptibility and prognosis. These tests are being done in conjunction with preceding histopathology for better results [16]. The telepathology helping the society and deals with obtaining, spreading, and broadcasting of histopathological pictures through the telecommunication networks viz. internet and satellite [17]. This practice will make the study of whole-slide easy and will let the prompt distributions of the images for early diagnosis and detail disease process.

Some commonly used histopathological techniques and stains in the developed countries routinely for diagnosis and the need of such methods and stains in the pathology set up of third world countries are.

6. Telepathy

It is basically the communication of thoughts among people without the use of common senses, which are specified for thinking, ideas and physical interaction purposes. This is being done without using body language or words. The main users/players of this technology is called mind readers or telepaths [18].

7. Digital pathology

This histologically based assessment revealed the lymphocytes that are infiltrating in the tumors as a substitute of the host immunity linked responses are being presented to be predictive and possibly chemopredictive in triple-negative and HER2-positive breast cancers. Though, the cooperation of the said lymphocytes, mediators, tumor cells, microenvironmental features, their quantity and associations are still awaiting to be explored. A tool named a digital pathology is anticipated to be used to evaluate the said features targeted and of chemotherapeutic reactions in patient. Based on digital pathology an image-analyzing algorithm are being developed to recognize lymphocytes, stromal, neoplastic cells in addition to obtaining of an image from the slides stained with H&E [19].

8. Multiplex immunohistochemistry

The prototype of molecular form of histopathology is fluctuating from a simple immunohistochemistry (single-marker) to multiplexed immunohistochemical recognition of markers to comprehend the multipart pathological procedures in an improved manner. This method is currently being used to explore the expression of those proteins pattern that is concerned in controlling of immune related checkpoints. In this histopathological technique the microarchitectural environment mapping of tumors is being done. This technique contributes in the understandings of syndrome heterogeneity and delivering all kinds of information you demand on time [20].

9. Immunofluorescence

This is a cell imaging technique and is being used commonly in laboratories. A fluorescent microscope is used in this technique and is run primarily for microbiological studies. The antibodies used in this method are conjugated chemically with fluorescent dyes which are then called labeled antibodies. These antibodies are later on attached to the specific cellular antigens. This largely valid method commonly practiced by the scientists to evaluate the localized and endogenous levels of protein and antigens expressions [21].

10. Brain mapping

Brain mapping is also including in the future of histopathology in which the positive and negative command is being generated in various segments of the brain. The technology used to detect the specified cortical regions of the brain during mapping is via very sensitive fMRI techniques [22].

11. Neuroimaging studies

It is a sort of new technique used for brain imaging. Through his technique the possible changes are visualized in the diseased brain. This technique is being used extensively in the infants and young babies. Because in young age the changes in the brain are being observed very rapid. The imaging techniques of the brain authorize a friendly procedure of neuro-receptor binding and neurophysiology. These imaging is sensitive and powerful tools for research purpose especially during pathophysiological studies of some foremost depressions. Currently, this practice is being used to observe the working capabilities of the brain and how the brain is fulfilling various major tasks including language processing [23].

Some commonly used histopathological stains in the developed countries routinely for diagnosis and the need of such stains in the pathology set up of third world countries are including as Stro-1 and vWF stains [24]; Simplified myeloperoxidase stain using benzidine dihydrochloride [25]; triphenyl tetrazolium chloride and tetrazolium red [26]; silver stain [27]; Giemsa, Diff3 and Warthin-Starry stains [28]; Gram and Steiner stains [29]; Toluidine blue, Masson's trichrome, Mallory's trichrome, Alcian blue. Reticulin, Azan, van Gieson, carmine, silver nitrate stains [1, 30].

Now most of the shortcomings are being overcome and the imminent archetype of histopathology is hypothesized to be digital in the near future. By this means the histopathologists will confirm diagnosis via virtual images analysis on computers instead of as usual morphometry and the digitized tissue could categorized into various histological grading for quantitative analysis, which results in provision of rapid and improved prospects for diagnosis and treatment of tumorous tissues.

Author details

Arbab Sikandar

Address all correspondence to: drarbab786@gmail.com

University of Veterinary and Animal Sciences, Lahore, Pakistan

References

[1] Bancroft JD, Stevens A. Theory and Practice of Histological Techniques. Edinburgh: Churchill-Livingstone; 1977. p. 129

[2] Sikandar A, Cheema AH, Adil M, Younus M, Zaneb H, Zaman A, Tipu MY, Masood S. Ovine paratuberculosis – A histopathological study from Pakistan. The Journal of Animal and Plant Sciences. 2013;**23**(3):749-753

[3] Young B, Woodford P, O'Dowd G. Wheater's Functional Histology E-Book: A Text and Colour Atlas. 6th Rev. ed. Elsevier Health Sciences. Churchill Livingstone, London.; 2013. p. 464

[4] Hench IB, Hench J, Tolnay M. Liquid biopsy in clinical management of breast, lung, and colorectal cancer. Frontiers in Medicine. 2018;**5**:9. DOI: 10.3389/fmed.2018.00009

[5] Sikandar A, Cheema AH, Younus M, Aslam A, Zaman MA, Rehman T. Histopathological and serological studies on paratuberculosis in cattle and buffaloes. Pakistan Veterinary Journal. 2012;**4**:547-551

[6] Luna D, Almerares A, Mayan 3rd JC, Gonzalez Bernaldo de Quiros F, Otero C. Health informatics in developing countries: Going beyond pilot practices to sustainable implementations: A review of the current challenges. Healthcare Informatics Research. 2014; **20**:3-10

[7] Bischofberger AS, Konar M, Ohlerth S, Geyer H, Lang J, Ueltschi G, Lischer CJ. Magnetic resonance imaging, ultrasonography and histology of the suspensory ligament origin: A comparative study of normal anatomy of Warmblood horses. Equine Veterinary Journal. 2006;**38**(6):508-516

[8] Cotran RS, Kumar V, Robbins SL. Robbins Pathologic Basis of Disease. Philadelphia: WB Saunders; 1989. pp. 39-86

[9] Sikandar A, Zaneb H, Younus M, Masood S, Aslam A, Ashraf S, Adil M, Rehman H. Protective effect of sodium butyrate on growth performance, immune responses and gut mucosal morphometry in salmonella-challenged broiler chickens. International Journal of Agriculture and Biology. 2017;**19**:1387-1393

[10] Subbarayappa BV. The roots of ancient medicine: An historical outline. Journal of Biosciences. 2001;**26**(2):135-143

[11] Culling CFA. Handbook of Histopathological and Histochemical Techniques: Including Museum Techniques. Oxford, United Kingdom: Butterworth-Heinemann; 2013

[12] Slaoui M, Fiette L. Histopathology procedures: From tissue sampling to histopathological evaluation. In: Drug Safety Evaluation. New York City: Humana Press; 2011. pp. 69-82

[13] Mathers CD, Loncar D. Projections of global mortality and burden of disease from 2002 to 2030. PLoS Medicine. 2006;**3**(11):e442

[14] Griffith LG, Naughton G. Tissue engineering – current challenges and expanding opportunities. Science. 2002;**295**(5557):1009-1014

[15] Saikia B, Gupta K, Saikia UN. The modern histopathologist: In the changing face of time. Diagnostic Pathology. 2008;**3**(1):25

[16] Aswathy MA, Jagannath M. Detection of breast cancer on digital histopathology images: Present status and future possibilities. Informatics in Medicine Unlocked. 2017;**8**:74-79

[17] Malami SA. Recent advances in telepathology in the developing world. In: Advances in Telemedicine: Applications in Various Medical Disciplines and Geographical Regions. London, United Kingdom: InTech; 2011

[18] Sorensen RA. Diary of a telepathic solipsist. Ratio. 2018;**31**(1):1-19

[19] Barnes M, Sarkar A, Redman R, Bechert C, Srinivas C. Development of a histology-based digital pathology image analysis algorithm for assessment of tumor infiltrating lymphocytes in HER2+ breast cancer. In: Cancer Research. Vol. 78, No. 4. Philadelphia, PA, USA: Amer Assoc Cancer Research; Feb 2018

[20] Gorris MA, Halilovic A, Rabold K, van Duffelen A, Wickramasinghe IN, Verweij D, Wortel IMN, Textor JC, Vries IJM de, Figdor CG, et al. Eight-color multiplex immunohistochemistry for simultaneous detection of multiple immune checkpoint molecules within the tumor microenvironment. The Journal of Immunology. 2018;**200**(1):347-354

[21] Lichtman JW, Conchello JA. Fluorescence microscopy. Nature Methods. 2005;**2**(12):910

[22] Jorge J, Figueiredo P, Gruetter R, van der Zwaag W. Mapping and characterization of positive and negative BOLD responses to visual stimulation in multiple brain regions at 7T. Human Brain Mapping. Feb 20. 2018

[23] Gernsbacher MA, Kaschak MP. Neuroimaging studies of language production and comprehension. Annual Review of Psychology. 2003;**54**(1):91-114

[24] Ning H, Lin G, Lue TF, Lin CS. Mesenchymal stem cell marker stro-1 is a 75 kd endothelial antigen. Biochemical and Biophysical Research Communications. 2011;**413**:353-357

[25] Kaplow LS, Ladd C. Brief report: Simplified myeloperoxidase stain using benzidine dihydrochloride. Blood. 1965;**26**(2):215-219

[26] Alexander MP. Differential staining of aborted and nonaborted pollen. Stain Technology. 1969;**44**(3):117-122

[27] Merril CR, Goldman D, Van Keuren ML. Gel protein stains: Silver stain. In: Methods in Enzymology. Vol. 104. Academic Press; 1984. pp. 441-447

[28] Genta RM, Robason GO, Graham DY. Simultaneous visualization of helicobacter pylori and gastric morphology: A new stain. Human Pathology. 1994;**25**(3):221-226

[29] Heilmann KL, Borchard F. Gastritis due to spiral shaped bacteria other than helicobacter pylori: Clinical, histological, and ultrastructural findings. Gut. 1991;**32**(2):137-140

[30] Alturkistani HA, Tashkandi FM, Mohammedsaleh ZM. Histological stains: A literature review and case study. Global Journal of Health Science. 2016;**8**(3):72-79. DOI: 10.5539/gjhs.v8n3p72

Chapter 2

Significance of Tumor Microenvironment Scoring and Immune Biomarkers in Patient Stratification and Cancer Outcomes

Kinan Drak Alsibai and Didier Meseure

Additional information is available at the end of the chapter

http://dx.doi.org/10.5772/intechopen.72648

Abstract

Tumors appear as heterogeneous tissues that consist of tumor cells surrounding by a tumor microenvironment (TME). TME is a complex network composed of extracellular matrix (ECM), stromal cells, and immune/inflammatory cells that drive cancer cells fate from invasion to intravasation and metastasis. The stromal-inflammatory interface represents a dynamic space, in which exchange of numerous molecular information is associated with the transition into tumorigenic microenvironment. Recruitment, activation, and reprogramming of stromal and immune/inflammatory cells in the extracellular space are the consequences of a reciprocal interaction between TME and cancer cells. Recent data suggest that cancer development is influenced by TME and controlled by the host's immune system, underlying the importance of TME components and immune biomarkers in the determination of prognosis and response to therapy. The immune classification has prognostic value and may be a useful supplement to the histopathological, molecular, and TNM classifications. Nevertheless, the complexity of quantitative immunohistochemistry and the variable assay protocols, stromal and immune cell types analyzed underscore the need to harmonize the quantified methods. It is therefore important to incorporate TME and immune scoring in determinations of cancer prognosis and to make sure they become a routine part of the histopathological diagnostic and prognostic assessment of patients.

Keywords: tumor microenvironment, stromal cells, immune cells, inflammatory cells, immunoscore, immune biomarkers, PDL-1, PD-1, checkpoint inhibitors, immuno-oncology, patient stratification, combined immunotherapy

1. Introduction

Cancer is usually viewed as a complex process of multiple disorders that are mostly driven by somatic mutation with the involvement of several hallmarks: genomic instability, sustaining proliferative signaling, resisting cell death, enabling replicative immortality, inflammation, evading the immune system, *de novo* angiogenesis, invasion, and metastasis. The outcome prediction in cancer is usually achieved by histopathological analysis of tissue samples obtained by biopsies or surgical specimens from primary tumor or metastatic localization. However, the heterogeneity in the histological appearance of different tumors (intertumor heterogeneity) as well as of different areas in the same tumor (intratumor heterogeneity) is of uncontested relevant and can explain the histopathological classification of tumors based on the morphological patterns. In the last decade, the advent of molecular pathology has allowed the definition of molecular subtyping for several cancers, which does not completely overlap with prevailing histopathological classifications [1].

In current practice, TNM classification appears as a sample method of tumor staging used worldwide, and based on tumor burden (T), lymph nodes status (N), and presence of metastases (M). However, the TNM classification provides limited prognostic information in cancer and does not predict response to therapy. Moreover, cancer outcome can differ significantly between patients whose cancers are at the same TNM stage.

Tumor appears as heterogeneous tissues that consist of tumor cells surrounded by a tumor microenvironment (TME). TME is a complex network composed of extracellular matrix (ECM), stromal cells (fibroblasts, adipocytes, neural and neuroendocrine (NE) cells, endothelial cells (ECs), and pericytes), immune and inflammatory cells that drive cancer cells fate from invasion to intravasation and metastasis. Cancer cells need cellular, biochemical, and biophysical stimuli originating from a more adapted microenvironment by recruiting and educating various types of normal cells into their neighborhood. The stromal-inflammatory interface represents a dynamic space characterized by reversible stromal and epithelial events. Within this dynamic space, exchange of numerous molecular information is associated with the transition into tumorigenic microenvironment and includes growth factors (GFs), cytokines, chemokines, enzymes, matrix proteins, and metabolic intermediates. Recruitment, activation, reprogramming, and persistence of stromal and immune/inflammatory cells in the extracellular space are the consequences of a reciprocal interaction between TME and cancer cells [2, 3].

Recent data suggest that cancer development is influenced by TME and controlled by the host's immune system, underlying the importance of including TME components and immunological biomarkers in the determination of prognosis and response to therapy, a concept that has been termed as microenvironment score and immunoscore. Increasingly, data collected from cancer tissue samples demonstrate that immune classification has prognostic value and may be a useful supplement to the histopathological, molecular, and TNM classifications. Nevertheless, the complexity of quantitative immunohistochemistry and the variable assay protocols, stromal and immune cell types analyzed and tumor-sampling criteria underscore the need to harmonize the quantified methods. It is therefore important to incorporate TME and immune scoring in determinations of cancer prognosis and to make sure they become a routine part of the histopathological diagnostic and prognostic assessment of patients with cancer.

2. Tumor microenvironment components

2.1. Non-immune/inflammatory stromal cells

Non-immune/inflammatory stromal cells comprise fibroblasts, adipocytes, neural and neuro-endocrine cells, endothelial cells, pericytes, and mesenchymal stem cells (MSCs) (**Figure 1** and **Table 1**).

2.1.1. Cancer-associated fibroblasts

Cancer-associated fibroblasts (CAFs) are a sub-population of activated fibroblasts with myo-fibroblastic phenotype that represent the predominant non-inflammatory stromal cell type in the TME. CAFs are heterogeneous cells of multiple origins, which are usually identified according to their different origins by expression of proteins such as mesenchymal biomarkers (vimentin and fibronectin), fibroblast-secreted protein-1 (FSP-1), α-smooth muscle actin (αSMA), tenascin-C, platelet-derived growth factor receptor (PDGFR), and fibroblast activation protein (FAP) [4, 5]. CAFs accumulation in the TME is often correlated with poor prognosis. They may promote tumor development and progression by promoting angiogenesis or by interacting with immune-inflammatory cells and neuroendocrine cells through different cell factors and cytokines [2]. CAFs may also hinder antitumor immune responses [4]. Indeed, cancer cells produce TGF-β that activates adjacent CAFs. In turn, CAFs promote tumor progression by releasing numerous interleukins (IL-1, IL-6, IL-8, and IL-22) and chemokines (CXC-chemokine ligand CXCL and CC-chemokine ligand CCL) [2]. CAFs can also secrete various chemotactic GFs (EGF, FGF, HGF PDGF, and VEGF), ECM proteins (collagens, fibronectins, tenascin C, and SPARC), enzymes such as matrix metalloproteinases (MMPs), lysyl oxidases (LOX) family, and cyclooxygenase 2 (COX2) [6].

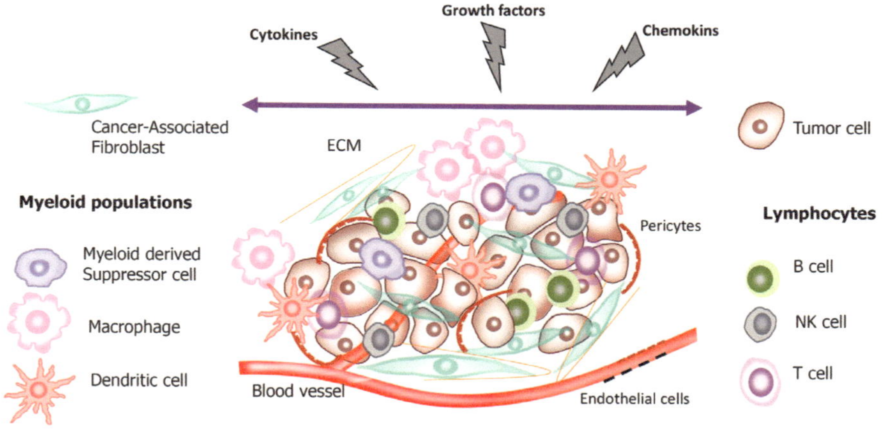

Figure 1. Tumor microenvironment is a complex network composed of extracellular matrix (ECM), stromal cells (fibroblasts, endothelial cells and pericytes) and immune and inflammatory cells (T cells, B cells, natural killer 'NK' cells, dendritic cells, macrophages and myeloid-derived suppressor cells). The stromal-inflammatory interface represents a dynamic space contains growth factors, cytokines and chemokines. Recruitment, activation, reprogramming and persistence of stromal and immune/inflammatory cells in the extracellular space are the consequences of reciprocal interactions between tumor microenvironment components and tumor cells.

Non-immune/ inflammatory stromal cell	Main markers	Main functions	Potential therapeutic targets
Cancer-associated fibroblasts (CAFs)	Vimentin, fibronectin, FSP-1, αSMA, tenascin-C, PDGFR Endosialin (CD248), and FAP	• Tumor progression (IL-1, IL-6, IL-8, IL-22, CXCL1 to CXCL12/ SDF1, CCL2 and CCL20, VEGF, PDGF, EGF, FGF, HGF, fibronectin, collagen I and III, EDA-fibronectin, tenascin C, SPARC, MMPs, LOX family, and COX2 • Promote angiogenesis • Hinder antitumor immune responses	Anti-CXCR-4 antibodies (CXCL12/SDF-1inhibition); anti-VEGF and anti-PDGF antibodies; MMP inhibitors; anti-IL6 antibodies; anti-HGF therapies; anti-FAP antibodies; Anti-TGFβ inhibitors; anti-IL-11 and anti-THSB1 therapies
Cancer-associated adipocytes (CAAs)	FSP-1 expression	• Produce adipokines (leptin, adiponectin, and apelin), angiogenic factors (VEGF), TNF-α, IL-1β, IL-6, IL-8, MCP1, CCL2 and CCL5 and HGF	Antibodies anti-IL-6, anti-IL-8; anti-CCL2, COX2 and adiponectin inhibitors
Mesenchymal stem cells (MSCs)	Vimentin, CD29 (β1integrin), CD44, CD73, CD90, CD105 and STRO-1	• Stimulate tumor angiogenesis through VEGF expression • Multilineage potentiate • Immunoregulatory function	Nano-engineered MSCs are used as targeted therapeutic carriers
Endothelial cells	Tip cells: $VEGFR1^{low}$, $VEGFR2^{high}$, $Dll4^{high,}$ and $CD34^{+}$ Stalk cells: $VEGFR1^{high}$, $VEGFR2^{low}$, $Dll4^{low}$ $CD34^{-}$.	• Implicated in metastatic niche and dormancy through TGF-β1 and POSTN	avβ1, avβ2, a5β1 integrin inhibitors; anti-VEGF and VEGFR agents
Pericytes	αSMA, Desmin, NG2 (CSPG4), 3G5 antigen, PDGFR-β and Endosialin (CD248)	• Modulate the magnitude of immune responses • Prevent lymphocyte extravasation and activation in tumor tissue	Anti-ANG2 antibody VEGFR and PDGFR-β antagonists; VEGFR, PDGFR-β, and Tie-2 agonists; anti-RSG5 and anti-PD/PD-L1 therapies
Neural cells	PGP9.5. and NGF	• Favors tumor progression • Norepinephrine, impact T-cells by inhibiting the generation of CTLs through inhibition of TNF-α synthesis	Anti-NGF blocking antibodies, NT3 and NT4 targeted therapies; GDNF inhibitors; anti-NGF antibodies; anti-PTN antibodies and N-syndecan inhibitors; BDNF inhibitors

Abbreviations: ANG2: angiopoietin-2; *Integrins* αv: avβ1, avβ2; BDNF: brain-derived neurotrophic factor; CCL: chemokine ligand; COX: cyclooxygenase; CSF: colony stimulating factor; CXCL: C-X-C chemokine ligand; CXCR: C-X-C chemokine receptor; CSPG4: Chondroitin sulfate proteoglycan 4; FAP: fibroblast activation protein; FRb: folate receptor beta; GDNF: glial cell line-derived neurotrophic factor; HRG: histadine-rich glycoprotein; IL: interleukin; MMP: matrix metalloproteinase; NGF: nerve growth factor; NT: neurotrophin; PDGF: platelet-derived growth factor; PDGFR: platelet-derived growth receptor; PD1: programmed cell death protein; PD-L1: programmed cell death ligand; PTN: pleiotropin; RSG5: regulator of protein signaling 5; SDF: stromal-derived factor; TIMP: tissue inhibitor of metalloproteinase; TGF: transforming growth factor; TLR: toll-like receptor; VEGF: vascular endothelial growth factor; VEGFR: vascular endothelial growth factor and receptor.

Table 1. Stromal cell types in tumor microenvironment: main markers and functions with potential therapeutic targets.

2.1.2. Cancer-associated adipocytes

Cancer-associated adipocytes (CAAs) possess important secretory properties that may enhance tumor aggressiveness. Compared to normal adipocytes, CAAs are characterized by the loss of adipocyte differentiation, a smaller size, and FSP-1 expression (with lack of αSMA expression). They produce adipokines (leptin, adiponectin, and apelin), angiogenic factors and GFs (VEGF and HGF), tumor necrosis factor-α (TNF-α), interleukins (IL-1β, IL-6, and IL-8), and chemokines (MCP1, CCL2, and CCL5) [7]. They also exhibit an increased secretion of fibronectin, collagen I/VI, and MMP-11/Stromelysin-3 [2, 8]. The activation of Wnt/β-catenin pathway in response to Wnt3a secreted by cancer cells is essential to adipocytes reprogramming. The reprogrammed CAAs located close to cancer cells can initiate protumoral heterotypic paracrine and endocrine interactions. Another type of CAAs is the adipose stem cells (ASCs). ASCs can influence the TME by worsening the tumorigenic behavior of c-Met-producing cancer cells, which in turn creates an inflammatory TME. ASCs can interact with TME through TGF-β1-signaling pathway or promote angiogenesis by migrating toward tumor-conditioned media through the PDGF-BB/PDGF-β-signaling pathway [5].

2.1.3. Angiogenic vascular cells

Blood vessels are composed of perivascular cells termed as pericytes, endothelial cells (ECs) which form the inner lining of the vessels wall and smooth muscle cells.

Pericytes differentiate from mesenchymal precursors and are recruited to tumors by PDGFβ. They possess characteristic cellular markers including 3G5 ganglioside and chondroitin sulfate proteoglycan 4 (CSPG4) also known as NG2. In tumor tissue, pericytes highly express αSMA, although it is often absent in quiescent pericytes in non-tumoral tissue. Recent experimental studies revealed that pericytes can actively modulate the magnitude of immune responses and may prevent lymphocyte extravasation and activation in tumor tissue [9].

ECs are subdivided into tip cells and stalk cells and function as active stromal regulators implicated in proliferation, invasion, secretion of inflammatory and growth mediators, and metastatic spread. Tip cell is highly migratory and polarized EC type that extends numerous filopodia and expresses low level of VEGF receptor 1 ($VEGFR1^{low}$), with high levels of VEGFR2 and Delta-like ligand 4 (Dll4), and in vitro CD34. The tip cell is followed by stalk cell, a proliferative and less migratory type of EC, which expresses $VEGFR1^{high}$, $VEGFR2^{low}$, $Dll4^{low}$ and has undetectable levels of CD34 in vitro [10]. Importantly, neovascular tips are rich in active TGF-β1 and periostin, which promote tumor growth and regulate tumor dormancy [11].

2.1.4. Neural and neuroendocrine cells

Cancer cells can support the neoneurogenesis by secreting several neuronal growth factors and axon guidance molecules. The majority of factors known to induce neurogenesis, such as neurotrophins, insulin-like growth factor-II (IGF-II), and fibroblast growth factor (FGF), are usually secreted by tumors with bad prognosis. These factors exert autocrine or paracrine effects in cancer cells. Norepinephrine, another neurotransmitter, has a significant impact on T-cells. It can inhibit the generation of antitumor cytotoxic T-lymphocytes (CTLs) through the inhibition of TNF-α synthesis [11]. The neural-epithelial interaction and nerve growth factor

(NGF) production by cancer cells favor tumor progression by promoting both the growth of cancer cells and neurites [12].

Neuroendocrine (NE) cells are part of the diffuse NE system and exhibit a combination of neuronal and endocrine features. NE system strongly influences the function of the immune system. It can regulate the migration and cytotoxicity in natural killer (NK) cells through neurotransmitters. Additionally, the neuroendocrine substance P (SP) blocks the β1-integrin-mediated adhesion of T lymphocytes and increases their migratory activity [13]. SP can also induce the production of various cytokines in leukocytes. SP and the subsequent activation of the neurokinin-1 receptor (NK1R) lead to mitogen-activated protein kinase (MAPK) activation. The involvement of NK1R activation in mitogenesis, angiogenesis, cell migration, and metastasis supports the hypothesis that SP and NK1R interactions influence the TME [14].

2.1.5. Mesenchymal stem cells

Mesenchymal stem cells (MSCs) are multipotent stem cells with the capacity to differentiate into fibroblasts, adipocytes, pericytes, osteocytes, and chondrocytes. MSCs express cell surface markers CD29, CD44, CD73, CD90, CD105, and STRO-1, and lack the expression of CD14, CD34, CD45, and human leukocyte antigen HLA-DR [15]. MSCs have immunomodulatory features and secrete cytokines, VEGF, and immune receptors which regulate the microenvironment in the host tissue. Based on their multilineage potentiate, immunoregulatory and tissue-protective properties, MSCs are being tested for the treatment and prevention of graft-versus-host disease, chronic diseases, and certain hematologic malignancies [16].

2.2. Extracellular matrix

ECM is composed of proteins (collagens, laminins, and fibronectins), proteoglycans, and hyaluronans in a specific organization [17, 18]. CAFs are the major cell type responsible for the synthesis of ECM proteins. ECM contains all the cytokines, GFs, and hormones secreted by stromal and cancer cells. During tumor progression, ECM composition and structure change continuously. ECM heterogeneity is crucial for controlling collective cell-invasive behaviors and determining metastasis efficiency. ECM selects survival cancer cells to aid in tumor growth and invasion at the fastest rate. ECM can also affect tumor development and metastasis through extracellular secretion, or by altering the phenotype of stromal cells or cancer cells [3]. Moreover, ECM provides a hypoxic or acidic microenvironment in which cancer cells have greater survival advantages. The abundant ECM within the TME is correlated with increased tumor growth through various mechanisms, including activation of pro-survival phosphoinositide 3-kinase (PI3K)-signaling pathways and downstream of integrin receptors [2].

ECM interacts with lymphocytes and crucially influences immune cells motility and localization, which can help tumor cells to evade from immune surveillance. Increased stroma density reduces lymphocyte displacement, supporting the idea that ECM deposition can alter antitumor immune responses by limiting T-cell motility [4].

2.3. Immune and inflammatory cells

Tumor microenvironment contains numerous immune and inflammatory cells that originate from lymphoid precursors [$CD8^+$ cytotoxic T-cells (CTLs), $CD45^+$ memory T-cells, $CD4^+$ T helper cells (Th1, Th2 and Th17), T regulatory cells (Tregs), T follicular helper cells (TFH), NKT cells, gamma delta T (γδ T) cells, B-cells, and plasmacytoid dendritic cells (pDCs)] and from myeloid precursors [tumor-associated macrophages (TAMs), myeloid-derived suppressor cells (MDSCs), conventional DCs (cDCs), neutrophils, mast cells, and platelets]. The term tumor-infiltrating lymphocytes (TILs) are referred to a group of T-cells (CD3, CD4, CD8, and FoxP3) located around tumor cells [19]. In addition, the invasive margins of cancers may comprise tertiary lymphoid structures (TLSs) that exhibit strong similarities with lymph node organization.

These immune and inflammatory cells infiltrate TME via a network of inflammatory chemotactic cytokines and chemokines produced by cancer cells.

NK cells ($CD56^+/CD3^-$) belong to the innate immune system and play an important role in protecting the host from infections and cancer. NKT cells ($CD56^+/CD3^+$) share a variety of markers for both T lymphocytes and NK cells. The γδ T-cells are an independent population of circulating lymphocytes that can sense pathogens. γδ T-cells can also induce DC maturation, functional activation and migration, and antigen presentation. NK, NKT cells, and γδ T-cells are present in TME in various cancer, and express the natural killer group 2D (NKG2D) receptor. NKG2D recognizes proteins encoded by the *MICA* and *MICB* locus, which are located within the major histocompatibility complex (MHC) on chromosome 6 near the *HLAB* locus [20].

$CD4^+$ and $CD8^+$ are the two main lineages of T-cells. $CD4^+$ T-cells are classified into CD4+ Th that mediate tumor immunity and $CD4^+$ $CD25^+$ $FoxP3^+$ Tregs that suppress antitumor immunity and promote tumor growth [21, 22].

DCs are derived from myeloid precursors (cDCs) or lymphoid precursors (pDCs) and are considered as a crucial link between innate and adaptive immunity. DCs have three maturation stages: precursor DCs, immature DCs, and mature DCs. Immature DCs interact with antigens, migrate into secondary lymphoid organs, and become antigen-presenting cells (APCs). DCs are among the first cells migrating to the tumor site by means of GFs (VEGF and HGF), chemokines (CXCL12 and CXCL8), and antimicrobial peptide (β-defensin) secreted by cancer cells and stromal cells [23–25].

MDSCs have two distinct monocytic and granulocytic subsets and can differentiate into DCs or ECs. They coordinate tumor progression and angiogenesis through the release of MMP-9 and VEGF. MDSCs can also promote immune evasion by suppressing antitumor CTLs and NK cells [26].

TAMs are multifunctional cells characterized by the expression of CD68, plasticity, and secretion of numerous immune-modulatory cytokines. Macrophages differentiation and growth are regulated by several GFs, including CSF-1 and GMCSF. TAMs can release chemokines (CCL17, CCL18, and CCL22) and recruit non-CTLs, especially Tregs. Activated macrophages can be classified into M1 and M2 cells [27]. M1 cells are characterized by high capacity to present antigen and are involved in the response of Th1 cells to pathogens and cancer. M1 cells produce proinflammatory cytokines (TNFα and IFN-γ) and interleukins (IL-1 and IL-12) and generate reactive oxygen species (ROS) and nitric oxide (NO). By contrast, M2 cells have immunosuppressive phenotype, produce IL-10, and inhibit CTLs, which are crucial to initiate a Th2-type response. Within the TME, TAMs have generally a M2-skewed phenotype ($CD163^+$, $CD204^+$, and $CD206^+$) that promote angiogenesis, ECM remodeling, and repair [28].

During tumor development, pre-invasive TME has antitumor property that includes predominantly M1 and Th1 with the production of IL-12, IFNγ, and inducible NO synthase (iNOS). Comparatively, the transition to invasive TME is marked by pro-tumoral properties with a shift from M1 to M2 and from Th1 to Th2 cells, a decrease of IFNγ, and an increase of IL-1, IL-6, VEGF, and indoleamine 2, 3-dioxygenase (IDO) [29].

Topographically, each type of immune and inflammatory cells has a preferred location within tumor site. CTLs and Th1 cells are located at the invasive margins and/or in the tumor core. Immature DCs are found in the tumor core, whereas mature DCs infiltrate T-cell zones in close contact with $CD4^+$ and $CD8^+$ T-cells. B-cells are found in TLS and at the invasive margins. TAMs and TFH are in contact or within B-cell zones, whereas NK cells are dispersed within the stroma and at the invasive margins [30].

Tumor-associated TLSs exhibit strong similarities with lymph node organization and comprise prominent B-cell follicles, T-cell marginal zones, and associated follicular DCs, very few Tregs, and high endothelial venules (HEVs). TLSs are usually located in the tumor-invasive margin and in the stroma of most cancers and their densities correlate with a favorable clinical outcome. HEVs express peripheral node addressins (PNAds) and specialized in the extravasation of circulating immune cells, and the secretion of chemokines that are crucial for lymphocyte recruitment and entry into the lymph node. Recently, a molecular signature of TLSs encoding 12 distinct chemokines (CCL2, CCL3, CCL4, CCL5, CCL8, CCL18, CCL19, CCL21, CXCL9, CXCL10, CXCL11, and CXCL13) has been identified in various tumors [31].

TLSs are associated with the generation of an adaptive immune response and represent a formidable school for T-cell priming, B-cell activation, and differentiation into plasma cells and an exquisitely located factory for antibody production [32].

3. Host immune response to cancer

3.1. Cancer immune cycle

In the early stage of carcinogenesis, cancer cells are rejected by an innate immune mechanism also referred to as immunosurveillance. The innate immune system recognizes exogenous pathogen-associated molecular patterns (PAMPs) or endogenous danger-associated molecular patterns (DAMPs). These latter ones are recognized by the host organism through various pattern recognition receptors (PRRs) that activate DNA sensors and downstream adaptors to trigger stimulation of innate immune system and to induce adaptive T-cell responses. Multiple families of PRRs, including Toll-like receptors (TLRs), have been identified within plasma membrane, intracellular vesicles, and within the cytosol of APCs [33]. Binding of ligands to PRRs activates various adaptor molecules and downstream signaling pathways, orchestrating innate immune responses and maturation of APCs (DCs), leading to production of antimicrobial peptides, cytokines, chemokines, and type I interferon (IFN) including IFN-α and IFN-β. In cancer, PRRs can also recognize various endogenous DAMPs, such as cancer-associated antigens (CAAs). Among regulators of innate immune system, recent evidence has indicated that the major pathway involved in the induction of a spontaneous antitumor adaptive T-cell response is the stimulator of interferon genes (STING) signaling [34].

Experimental studies indicate that immune system plays a dual role in cancer, a theory known as cancer immunoediting. It can not only eliminate cancer cells or inhibit their growth but also promote tumor progression by modifying conditions within TME or by selecting more resistant cancer cells. Cancer immunoediting contains three phases: elimination, equilibrium, and escape. The immune system is directed against cancer cells through the "cancer immunity cycle" described by Chen and Mellman [35], which associates cancer antigen release by tumor cells, presentation by DCs and priming of T lymphocytes in lymph nodes, activation of peripheral immune cells, trafficking and infiltration of T-cells to the TME, cancer cells recognition, and immune-mediated cell death (T-cell-inflamed phenotype). In the elimination phase, T-cells attack tumor cells that express tumor-specific antigens in the form of complexes of tumor-derived peptides bound to MHC molecules on the cell. Naïve T-cells that differentiate in bone marrow express a unique T-cell receptor (TCR) and undergo positive and negative selection processes in thymus. T-cells become activated when tumor antigens are recognized. Then, T-cells proliferate and differentiate, leading to the T-cell's ability to attack and destroy cells that express relevant antigens. The recognition of antigen-MHC complexes by the T-cell antigen receptor is not sufficient for the activation of naïve T-cells. However, the engagement of CD28 on T-cell surface and the expression of B7 molecules (CD80 and CD86) on APCs (DCs) provide additional costimulatory signals [36]. Cancer cells usually do not express B7 molecules (except for certain lymphomas) and hence are largely invisible to the immune system. This can be overcome by an inflammatory response, which permits APCs to take up antigen and present antigen-MHC along with B7 molecules initially in tumor-draining lymph nodes for effective activation of T-cells. After the costimulation process, tumor-specific T-cells acquire effector function, move to the tumor site, and infiltrate TME, which activates the antitumor immune response. However, the antitumor efficacy of T-cells within TME is determined by their ability to overcome barriers and counter-defenses they encounter from tumor and stromal cells, Tregs, MDSCs, and inhibitory cytokines that act to mitigate antitumor immune responses [37].

Activated T-cells express immune checkpoints such as cytotoxic T lymphocyte-associated protein 4 (CTLA-4 also known as CD152) and programmed death 1 (PD-1 also known as CD279) which act to abrogate T-cells responses. CTLA-4 competes with CD28 for binding to CD80/86, providing an inhibitory stimulus upon engagement [38].

PD-1 is a T-cell surface receptor that delivers inhibitory signals upon engagement with its ligands. PD-1 ligands (PD-L1 and PD-L2) are expressed via oncogenic expression on tumor cells or by stromal cells and may also be upregulated in the setting of high levels of IFN-γ, termed adaptive immune resistance [39].

During tumor development, a subpopulation of non-immunogenic cancer cells develops new mechanisms to evade immune surveillance and induce tumor tolerance. They include decreased expression of MHC-I and expression of immunosuppressive factors that contribute to escape from immune recognition. Consequently, tumors display a strong immune-suppressive TME and fail to elicit an appropriate adaptive immune response. This TME is associated with several molecular mechanisms in place to interfere with CTLs, resulting in poor infiltration of reactive tumor-rejecting T-cells [40].

After an efficient immune response, immune tolerance reduces ability for immune-mediated tumor eradication by associating upregulation of tumor and immune cells PD-L1, DCs and macrophages IDO expression in response to IFNγ signaling, expression of additional immunosuppressive checkpoints (LAG3), and enhanced regulatory T-cells and MDSCs activities [41].

An innate immune response leads to activation of the adaptive immune system (B- and T-cells), provided direct interactions with APCs and a proinflammatory environment. Primary adaptive responses are slower than the innate responses, as clonal expansion due to the recognition of foreign antigens is required.

The current understanding of the dichotomous nature of immune cells in tumors is that IFN-γ-producing $CD4^+$ Th1 and $CD8^+$ CTL along with mature DCs, NK cells, M1 macrophages and type 1 NKT cells can generate antitumor responses. Conversely, $CD4^+$ Th2, $CD4^+$ Tregs, MDSCs, immature DCs, M2 macrophages, and type 2 NKT cells promote tumor tolerance and support tumor growth and progression [40]. Furthermore, the knowledge on the crucial antitumor activity of the immune system has generated great interest in immunotherapy of cancer, including non-immunogenic tumors.

3.2. Humoral immune response in cancer

The production of autoantibodies (AAbs) reflects the immunologic reactivity in cancer patients and enhances immune surveillance for cancer cells. AAbs level is detectable in very early cancer stages and may persist for an extended period after cancer removal, reflecting the overall host immune response toward the tumor. It is interesting to note that a repertoire of AAbs is shared by autoimmune diseases and cancer, suggesting that autoimmune conditions share many parallels with the humoral immune response to tumor-associated antigens (TAAs) [42]. Tolerance defects, inflammation, posttranslational modifications, and cell death can affect TAA immune presentation, contributing to cancer-related AAbs production. Recently, AAbs have become useful diagnostic, prognostic, and surveillance cancer biomarkers as they can be easily detected in the serum of cancer patient [43].

3.3. Genetic and germline polymorphisms of immune system

Genetic polymorphism is an alternative phenotype that appears to be widespread among the genes of the immune system and can correspond to an evolutionary adaptation of the host organism facing an environment in constant evolution. Several polymorphisms concerning genes that encode Janus kinase/signal transducer and activator of transcription (JAK/STAT), *TLR* genes, TNF-α, NF-κB, NOD2, autophagy-related protein 16 (ATG16), and receptors for the Fc domain of immunoglobulins (FcR), are involved in the immune responses in cancer development or affect the potency of certain anticancer therapies.

JAK/STAT-signaling pathway plays a key role in the regulation of cellular responses to cytokines (IFN-α, IFN-β, IFN-γ, and IL). It has been demonstrated that genetic polymorphism involved in JAK/STAT (STAT3 and STAT4) pathway is associated with the risk of non-Hodgkin lymphoma [44]. Moreover, polymorphisms in *TLR* genes may shift balance between pro- and anti-inflammatory cytokines in the host, contributing to the onset and progression of cancers. Recent evidence has implicated polymorphisms of FcRs in the efficacy of monoclonal antibody (mAb)-mediated therapy. Interestingly, the therapeutic effects of IgG1 mAbs (rituximab and trastuzumab) are partially mediated by the FcγR immune response, suggesting that polymorphisms of FcγRs may affect the potency of the mAb treatment [45].

3.4. Microbiota

The microbiota is composed of commensal bacteria and other microorganisms that live on the epithelial barriers of the host. Microbiota influences physiological functions including the maintenance of barrier homeostasis and the regulation of metabolism, hematopoiesis, inflammation, and immunity. Recent data demonstrated the involvement of microbiota in cancer initiation, progression, and dissemination. In addition, gut microbiota can modulate the response to chemotherapy, radiotherapy and immunotherapy, and susceptibility to toxic side effects. Therefore, targeting the microbiota may improve anticancer efficacy and prevent toxicity [46].

3.5. Environmental factors

Immunity in humans can also be affected by environmental factors, including the presence of infectious agents, diet, exposure to sunlight (photoimmunity), and the intake of pharmaceuticals. Interestingly, during periods of decreased exposure to sunlight the human immune responses are associated with enhanced levels of IL-6 and C-reactive protein, which are linked to an increased propensity for autoimmunity. Therefore, it is acceptable to believe that low sunlight conditions may correlate with a more inflammatory systemic environment, leading to better responses to cancer immunotherapy [47].

4. Tumor microenvironment and immune scoring

4.1. Glasgow microenvironment score

Glasgow microenvironment score (GMS) is a cumulative prognostic score that combines Klintrup-Mäkinen (K-M) grade and tumor stroma percentage (TSP) and has an independent prognostic value. K-M grade semiquantitatively evaluates the peritumoral immune cell type and density at the invasive margin of the deepest point of tumor invasion using H&E-stained FFPE tissues. K-M grade is classified into (1) low-grade K-M: no increase or mild increase in inflammatory cells, and (2) high-grade K-M: prominent inflammatory reaction that forms a band at the invasive margin, or florid cup-like infiltrate at the invasive edge with destruction of cancer cell islands [48, 49]. K-M grade could be assessed by IHC-stained sections using CD3, CD8, CD45R0, and FoxP3 antibodies to evaluate immune T-cell type [49]. TSP evaluates the percentage of stroma using complete sections of the deepest point of tumor invasion. The proportion of stroma is calculated as the visible field at 10× objective, excluding areas of mucin and/or necrosis [50]. TPS is subsequently graded as low TSP (≤50%) or high TSP (>50%) [49]. The global GMS score is subdivided into three GMS categories: (GMS 0: high-grade K-M), (GMS 1: low-grade K-M/low-grade TSP), and (GMS 2: low-grade K-M/high-grade TSP) [51].

4.2. Microenvironment cell populations-counter

Microenvironment cell populations (MCP)-counter is a transcriptome-based computational method that quantifies the abundance of 10 stromal and immune cell populations in TME using a single-gene expression experiment. MCP-counter produces an abundance score for $CD3^+$ T-cells (CD3D and CD5), CD8+ (CD8B) and CTLs (EOMES and GNLY), B lymphocytes (CD19, CD79A, and CD79B), NK cells (NKp46 and KIR genes), monocytic lineage (CSF1R), myeloid DCs (CD1), neutrophils (FCGR3B and CD66b), as well as fibroblasts (DCN and TAGLN) and ECs (CDH5). These scores can then be used for direct comparisons of the abundance of the corresponding cell type across samples within a cohort. MCP-counter was quantitatively validated by both using mRNA mixtures and IHC in FFPE tissues. This method can reproduce immunological and stromal prognostic classifications associated with overall survival in lung adenocarcinoma and colorectal and breast cancers [52]. However, the loss of spatial cell's localization is one of limitations when using such transcriptomic technology. Thus, histological confirmation of MCP-counter seems to be necessary in cases where contamination of samples by surrounding non-tumoral tissues is unavoidable.

4.3. Cancer transcriptomic signature

A transcriptomic classification of colorectal cancer has been recently proposed that stratifies colorectal cancer into intrinsic subtypes with different prognosis. This classification is subdivided into four consensus molecular subtypes (CMS): CMS1 (MSI-like subtype) that contains most microsatellite instability (MSI) tumors and BRAF mutations, CMS2 (canonical subtype) with high chromosomal instability (CIN), CMS3 (metabolic subtype) includes tumors with KRAS mutations and shows a disruption of metabolic pathways, and CMS4 (mesenchymal subtype) that concerns tumors with frequent CpG-island methylator phenotype (CIMP) [53]. Interestingly, a recent comparative study has demonstrated three microenvironmental signatures that correspond to each molecular subtype. The CMS1 was associated with the overexpression of genes specific to cytotoxic lymphocytes, and a good prognosis. Conversely, CMS4 revealed proinflammatory, proangiogenic, and immunosuppressive signature and was associated with poor prognosis. Finally, CMS2 and CMS3 showed almost similar TME profile and were associated with low immune and inflammatory signatures, and intermediate prognosis [54] (**Table 2**).

Comparatively, in triple-negative breast cancer, three TME subtypes using IHC analyses have been identified: (1) a first subtype with $TLR9^{high}$ expression by cancer cells, hypercellular stroma and numerous TILs overexpressing TLR9; (2) a second subtype with $TLR9^{low}$ expression by cancer cells, a predominantly paucicellular stroma, and rare inflammatory cells expressing TLR9 without TILs; and (3) a third subtype with $TLR9^{low}$ expression by cancer cells, a predominantly fibrotic and vascular stroma containing some immune and inflammatory cells [55].

4.4. Tumor microenvironment of metastasis score

Tumor microenvironment of metastasis (TMEM) score is an IHC-staining score assessed by three antibodies: anti-CD31, anti-CD68, and anti-panMena. The selected area should be identified by low power, focusing on representative high density and adequacy of tumor, and lack of necrosis, inflammation, and artifacts. TMEM is defined as a structure composed of the direct

Consensus molecular subtypes (CMS)		Molecular characteristics [53]	MCP-counter signature [54]	Mechanisms of action	Prognosis
CMS1	MSI-like subtype	• MSI tumors with mutations in genes encoding DNA mismatch-repair proteins, resulting in high mutational burden • Tumors with a CIMP and BRAF mutations	Overexpression of genes specific to cytotoxic lymphocytes	High expression of genes coding for T-attracting chemokines (CXCL9, CXCL10, and CXCL16) or TLS's formation (CXCL13), Th1 cytokines IFNG and IL15	Good prognosis
CMS2	Canonical subtype	• Tumors with high chromosomal instability • Activation of the Wnt and MYC pathways	Low immune and inflammatory signatures		Intermediate prognosis
CMS3	Metabolic subtype	• Tumors with KRAS mutations and disruption of metabolic pathways	Low immune and inflammatory signatures		Intermediate prognosis
CMS4	Mesenchymal subtype	• Tumors with mesenchymal phenotype and frequent CIMP phenotype	Expression markers of lymphocytes and of cells of monocytic origin. Proinflammatory, proangiogenic, and immunosuppressive signature	High expression of myeloid chemokine CCL2, complement components, angiogenic factors (VEGFB, VEGFC, and PDGFC), and immunosuppressive molecules (TGFB1, TGFB3, LGALS1, and CXCL12)	Poor prognosis

Table 2. Cancer transcriptomic signature: molecular subtypes versus tumor microenvironment signature.

contact between an invasive pan Mena-overexpressing carcinoma cell, an endothelial cell ($CD31^+$), and a perivascular macrophage ($CD68^+$), with no discernible stroma between tumor cell and perivascular macrophage. Then, the number of TMEMs per 10 high-power fields (×400) is calculated to give a final TMEM score for each patient sample [56, 57]. In breast cancer, TMEM score is positively associated with risk of distant metastasis in $ER^+/HER2^-$ patients [57].

4.5. Recommendations for assessing TILs in breast cancer

A group of experts has proposed a step-by-step recommendation of how TILs should be evaluated by pathologists in breast carcinoma tissue samples [58], whether it can be on core biopsies or full surgical sections:

- One section (4–5 μm, magnification × 200–400) per patient is considered to be sufficient.
- Full sections are preferred over biopsies whenever possible.
- TILs should be evaluated within the borders of the invasive tumor.

- TILs should be reported as percentage for the stromal compartment (percentage of stromal TILs).
- TILs should be assessed as a continuous parameter. The percentage of stromal TILs is a semiquantitative parameter for this assessment, for example, 80% stromal TILs means that 80% of the stromal area shows a dense mononuclear infiltrate.
- All mononuclear cells (including lymphocytes and plasma cells) should be scored, but polymorphonuclear leukocytes are excluded.
- Do not focus on hotspots: a full assessment of average TILs in the tumor area should be used.
- Exclude TILs outside of the tumor border and around DCIS and normal lobules.
- Exclude TILs in tumor zones with crush artifacts, necrosis, regressive hyalinization as well as in the previous core biopsy site.

4.6. PDL-1/TILs score

Tumors can be classified into four groups based on their PD-L1 expression and the presence or absence of TILs [59, 60] (**Table 3**). The type of tumors that fit into each of PD-L1/TILs status depends on the genetic aberrations and oncogene drivers of these tumors. In melanoma, a high proportion of type I (~38%) and type II (~41%) tumors is observed, with the former having considerably the best prognosis [59]. Comparatively, pancreatic cancer has a lower level of PD-L1 expressed on tumor and immune cells [61]. By contrast, in non-small-cell lung cancer (NSCLC) where the oncogenes are more important drivers of tumor PD-L1 expression, the frequency of type III may be higher. In NSCLC, PD-L1 positivity is associated to adenocarcinoma and the presence of EGFR mutations, whereas PD-1 is associated with smoking status and the presence of KRAS mutations [62]. Additionally, increased levels of CD3 and $CD8^+$ are associated with better outcome in NSCLC [63].

Accumulating data suggest that two major categories of immune resistance within the TME may exist: (i) failure of T-cell trafficking due to low levels of inflammation and lack of chemokines for migration, and (ii) dominant suppression through immune-inhibitory mechanisms. The potential reasons explaining failed tumor rejection in the cases of T-cell-inflamed TME include extrinsic inhibition by PD-L1/PD-1 interactions and the suppression effect of Tregs [64].

Expression groups	PDL-L1/TILs status	Significations
Group I	PD-L1+, with presence of TILs	Drives adaptive immune resistance
Group II	PD-L1−, with no TIL	Indicates immune ignorance
Group III	PD-L1+, with no TIL	Indicates intrinsic induction
Group IV	PD-L1−, with presence of TILs	Indicates the role of other suppressor in promoting immune tolerance

Table 3. PDL-1/TILs score: tumors can be classified into four groups based on their PD-L1 expression and presence or absence of TILs.

4.7. PD-L1 tumor proportion score

Immunotherapies with checkpoint inhibitor PD-L1, which can inhibit T-cell function by binding PD-1 on T-cells, have shown encouraging results in patients with advanced NSCLC. Several agents such as pembrolizumab, nivolumab, atezolizumab, and durvalumab are approved or under clinical development for patients with metastatic NSCLC. Clinical trials have shown an association between the degree of clinical efficacy of these drugs and the level of PD-L1 expression by IHC. In two recent comparative trials, at least three PD-L1 IHC antibodies (22C3, 28–8, and SP263) are aligned regarding PD-L1 expression on tumor cells [65, 66]. A cancer cell is considered PD-L1 positive only when cell membrane is partially or completely stained. By contrast, an immune cell is considered PD-L1 positive if it features any PD-L1 staining: cell membrane or cytoplasm. PD-L1-positive immune cells are predominantly macrophages and lymphocytes. All assays revealed PD-L1 expression on immune cells, but with greater variance than expression on tumor cells. Alveolar macrophages are consistently stained with anti-PD-L1 antibody, serving as an internal positive control.

In NSCLC, PD-L1 tumor proportion score (TPS) is proposed to evaluate the IHC expression on tumor cells. The cutoffs of the different scoring criteria may be integrated into a six-step scoring system (Cologne Score: <1, ≥1, ≥5, ≥10, ≥25, ≥50%).

Currently, pathologists are confronted with two situations to evaluate TSP:

First-line metastatic NSCLC: Pembrolizumab is indicated in first-line setting as both monotherapy and combination therapy in metastatic NSCLC, which has TPS of ≥50%, with no EGFR or ALK genomic aberrations [67].

Second-line metastatic NSCLC: Pembrolizumab is indicated in second-line treatment of metastatic or locally advanced NSCLC, which has PD-L1 TPS of ≥1%. In this case, patients with EGFR or ALK genomic aberrations should have disease progression on therapy for these aberrations prior to receiving Pembrolizumab [61].

The above-cited data underline the importance of PD-L1 test as a biomarker in immunotherapy of NSCLC even in the first-line treatment. Nevertheless, the priority remains to harmonize the procedure of PD-1 testing and interpretation, which might require specific standardization. Therefore, pathologists have a major role to put in place the PDL-1 IHC test in routine practice and determine PDL-1 immunoscore on FFPE tissues.

5. Strategy panels in immunotherapy

Systemic anticancer therapies have evolved from chemotherapy through targeted therapies to immune agents and immunotherapy, which is now considered as the third paradigm in cancer treatment. Events from cancer immunity cycle and immune tolerance may serve as both predictive biomarkers and potential therapeutic targets. Immunotherapy is emerging as a novel therapeutic strategy promoting immune response against cancer cells and differing from traditional modalities that target tumor cells directly. Preclinical and clinical evidence provides the rationale for different promising immunotherapeutic approaches combining upregulation of immune responses and downregulation of immune tolerance, to edify a cancer immunity cycle or to re-activate a neutralized preexisting anticancer immune response [68].

Immunotherapies are most effective in patients with a T-cell-inflamed phenotype. Initially, immunotherapy using high-dose interleukin 2 and adoptive T-cell transfer allowed durable clinical benefit in patients with advanced malignancies. Currently, immune strategies have shifted to targeted manipulation of immune checkpoints. Immune checkpoints refer to multiple inhibitory and costimulatory pathways that counteract certain crucial steps of T-cell-mediated immunity to maintain self-tolerance and modulate the duration and amplitude of immune responses. Immune checkpoints are initiated primarily through T-cell inhibiting and stimulating receptors and their ligands, including CTLA-4 (CD152), PD-1 (CD279) and PD-L1 (CD274) or PD-L2 (CD273), among many others [41]. The CTLA-4 antibody ipilimumab was the first approved checkpoint inhibitor after it improved overall survival in patients with advanced melanoma in two randomized phase III trials. However, objective responses are low with ipilimumab monotherapy and 22% of patients with advanced melanoma survived at least 3 years after therapy. Greater clinical benefit has been observed with inhibitors targeting PD-1 or PD-L1 checkpoints. The anti-PD-1 inhibitors pembrolizumab and nivolumab have been recently approved by the US Food and Drug Administration (FDA) for patients with advanced unresectable melanoma, NSCLC, and metastatic renal-cell carcinoma, with objective responses in 40–45, 20, and 25% of patients, respectively. FDA approvals have been announced for nivolumab in patients with refractory Hodgkin's lymphoma and for the anti-PD-L1 agent atezolizumab in patients with advanced bladder cancer. Furthermore, significant clinical benefit, including durable tumor responses and extension of progression-free and overall survival, has now been observed with other anti-PD-1 and anti-PD-L1 inhibitors in a wide spectrum of solid tumors and hematological malignancies [69, 70].

However, significant responses to immunotherapy only occur in a minority of patients. Attempts are being made to improve the activity of immunotherapies with novel combinatorial strategies and with biomarker optimization. Immuno-oncology drugs are thus currently evaluated and data from recent clinical phase I–III trials have highlighted the potential for combination therapies, including these immunomodulating inhibitory molecules (TIM-3, VISTA, LAG-3, IDO, and KIR) and costimulatory antibodies (CD40, GITR, OX40, CD137, ICOS) [41, 71, 72].

6. Biomarkers in immuno-oncology

Selection of patients based on validated predictive biomarkers is an important issue that needs to be addressed. Although most of immunotherapies are dedicated to T lymphocytes and cell-mediated cytotoxicity, cancer immune response is a very complex process characterized by numerous reciprocal interactions between tumor cells, multiple immune/stromal cellular subtypes, soluble mediators, ECM, and blood vessels. A wide spectrum of biomarkers is thus required to guide anticancer immune strategies. Immunotherapeutic agents function through different mechanisms of action, including modulation of T-cell receptors (CTLA-4 and PD-1) and adoptive T-cell therapies that associate TILs, chimeric antigen receptors (CARs), and TCR-modified T-cells. Furthermore, tumor spatio-temporal heterogeneity is characterized by different antigenic profiles over time (before and after treatment) and topography (primitive and metastatic tumor) and numerous immunosuppressive mechanisms are promoted in the TME. Most importantly, discovering and optimizing immuno-oncology biomarkers could predict sensitivity or resistance to these immunomodulating molecules, identify their mechanisms of action, and define efficient combined therapies to rationally select patients. Thus, characterizing the anticancer immune response with multidisciplinary and multiparametric NGS and in situ technologies is pivotal to identify multiplex profiles that could allow patient's stratification for optimal personalized immunotherapy [73].

According to the thematic hallmarks of anticancer immune response, a large spectrum of potential biomarkers that could predict response to immunotherapy have been recently identified, including (i) tumor foreignness: tumor immunogenicity, high mutational load, gene expression profiling, epigenetic modifications of immune genes, intra-tumor heterogeneity; (ii) immunosuppressive tumor metabolism: LDH and TGFβ levels; (iii) host immune status: total lymphocyte count, T-cell and B-cell repertoire, antitumor antibodies titers, preexisting autoimmunity; (iv) immune regulation: antigen presentation (CD40/CD40L), cancer cells reduced MHC expression, T-cell recognition, TCR repertoire diversity, IFNα and TNFα levels; (v) immune cells migration: T-cell trafficking chemokines (CCL5, CXCL9, and CXCL10), chemokines profile, VEGF levels, inflammatory signature; (vi) tumor immune infiltration: $CD8^+$ TILs, FoxP3+ Tregs; (vii) T-cell cytotoxicity: granzyme A, perforin 1, and IFNγ levels; and (viii) immunosuppressive molecules: CTLA4, PDL1, PDL2, LAG3, TIM3, and IDO [73, 74].

These multiple predictive biomarkers present potential great interest in future practice to select patients for optimal immunotherapy: (i) PD-L1 expression in the TME may indicate increased sensibility to PD-1/PD-L1 checkpoint inhibitors; (ii) the presence of TILs suggests a preexisting antitumor immune response that can be reinitialized by immunotherapy; (iii) high tumor mutational load and neoantigens may be indicative of high tumor immunogenicity and sensitivity to immunotherapy; and (iv) the presence of immunosuppressive cells (immature DCs, MDSCs, TAMs, and Tregs), polarization of macrophages (anti-inflammatory M2 macrophages) and DCs (immunosuppressive/tolerogenic regulatory DCs), immunosuppressive molecules and immunoinhibitory cytokines may predict resistance to immunotherapy [72, 75].

Currently, only PD-L1 IHC assays have been validated for clinical utility, although several tumors, host, and environmental biomarkers are very promising candidate for patients' stratification. NGS and in situ technologies investigating tumor-immune interactions include multiplex immunohistochemistry (multiplexed-IHC), whole-exome sequencing (WES), transcriptome analysis, proteomics, and flow cytometry. However, before clinical application, each of these potential biomarkers requires high-quality validation process, comprising assessment of basic assay performance, characterization of the performance of the assay, and validation in clinical trials.

Recent technological advances have provided new tools that will facilitate an in-depth understanding of the interaction between the immune system and tumor cells, particularly in the TME and will help guide the development of personalized cancer immunotherapies. Data generated from these innovative technologies (i.e., gene microarray, deep-sequencing technologies, mass cytometry, and multicolor IHC staining) are classified into three categories: (i) function (to evaluate the function of different immune cells), (ii) phenotype (to provide the frequency and status of these cells), and (iii) signature/pattern (to elucidate the potential mechanisms of action) [76].

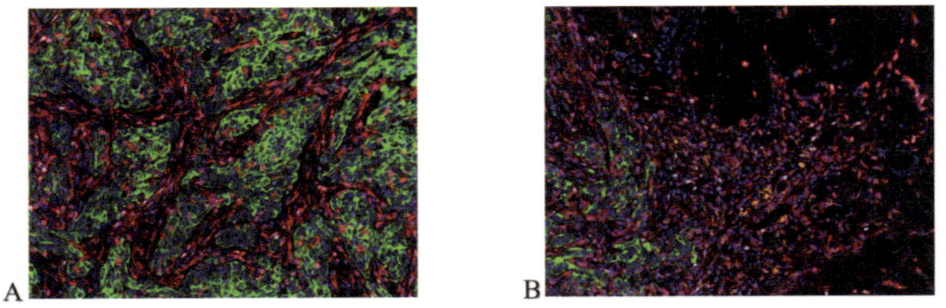

Figure 2. Fluorescent multiplex immunohistochemistry. (A) Breast cancer, section from tumor's core, and (B) section from invasive margin of the same tumor. The sections are stained with cytokeratin (cancer cells, in green), CD45RO (memory lymphocytes, in red), CD4 (T helper cells, in orange) and FoxP3 (in blue).

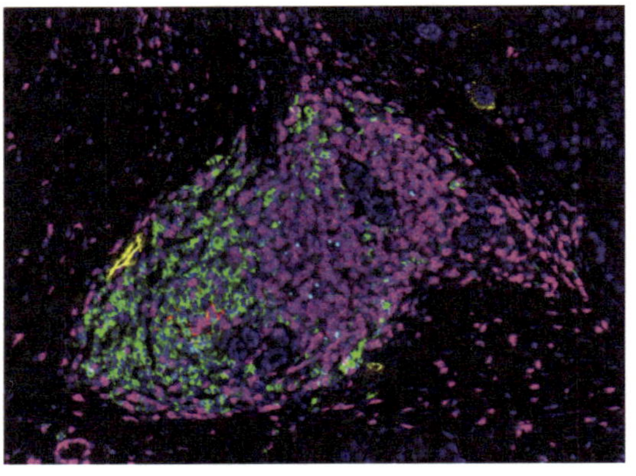

Figure 3. Fluorescent multiplex immunohistochemistry. Tertiary lymphoid structure panel stained with CD20 (B cells, in green), CD3 ($CD3^+$ T lymphocytes, in purple), DC-Lamp (mature DCs, in blue), CD21 (follicular DCs) and PNAd (high endothelial venule, in yellow).

Among these novel technologies, multiplex immunohistochemistry (multiplexed-IHC) appears as very effective and efficient method to identify on the same section and at the same time, several immune cell types, their location, and their state of activation, as well as the presence of immunoactive molecular expression. Multiplexed-IHC is a quantitative, image analysis-based method, using multicolor IHC on FFPE tissues, automated multispectral slide imaging, and advanced recognition software. When coupled with fluorophores (fluorescence multiplexed-IHC), this method takes advantage of light emission with different spectral peaks against a dark background (**Figures 2A**, **B** and **3**). Fluorescence multiplexed IHC provides spatial localization and distribution of phenotypic and functional biomarkers within the TME and thus is highly beneficial in experimental research for exploring immune evasion mechanisms or finding potential biomarkers [77].

7. Conclusion and perspectives

After chemotherapy and targeted therapy, immunotherapy has become the third paradigm in cancer. Immunotherapy is a key component of the therapeutic strategies to control and

http://dx.doi.org/10.5772/intechopen.72648

potentially cure cancer. The complexity and heterogeneity of the interaction between the immune system and tumor cells, particularly in the tumor microenvironment, underlies the immune status (i.e., immunologically responsive or immunologically ignorant) of each tumor for every patient. These reciprocal interactions depend on the organ, the oncogenic processes, and their modification by treatments. Although immunomodulation by checkpoint inhibitors (targeting both CTLA-4 and the PD-1/PD-L1 axis) induced a durable tumor response in several malignancies, the use of PD-L1 immunohistochemistry alone has not been sufficient for ruling in or out the use of anti-PD-1 or anti-PD-L1 expression-based therapies. Therefore, characterization of recognized tumor antigens, effector T-cell function, and immune-suppressive mechanisms, TILs, T-cell receptor repertoire, and mutational or neoantigen burden should be aimed at creating an optimized model for predicting response to anti-PD-1 or anti-PD-L1 therapies. Furthermore, specific mechanisms of T-cell exclusion such as activation of the WNT/β-catenin-signaling pathway, microbiota status, and genetic polymorphism should be included in future biomarker development (**Table 4**).

Accumulating evidences support that the optimal strategy for further immunotherapy development is combinatory regimens. The challenge of increasing the curative immune responses in a diverse population of patients will require multiple complementary therapeutic modalities to overcome the immunosuppressive tumor microenvironment. Thus, understanding the tumor microenvironment may offer opportunities to predict response to therapy and select the most appropriate immunotherapy for each patient. The recent availability of high-throughput next-generation sequencing and in situ technologies to quantify the different elements of the tumor microenvironment and understand their functionality opens the way for generalization of these approaches and the subsequent application of precision-personalized therapies based on these landscapes rather than on cancer subtypes only.

Stratification factors	**Tumor microenvironment subtypes**			**Cancer immune set point**
Morphology	**Immune/ inflammatory**	**Mesenchymal**	**Paucicellular/ inactive**	
Immunophenotype	**Immune response**	**Immune exclusion**	**Immune desert**	
Biological mechanisms	Tumor infiltration by cytotoxic T-cells, B-cells, MDSCs, NK cells regulatory T-cells, CAFs	Stromal-based inhibition from vessels, ECM, chemokines	Absence of preexisting antitumor immunity (ignorance, tolerance, no priming of T-cells)	
Biomarkers				
Tumor genome/epigenome				
Tumor mutation load	High	Low	Low	Positive effect
Neoantigen burden	High	Low	Low	Positive effect
Gene expression profiling	Activation signature^{high}	Activation signature^{low}	Activation signature$^{very\ low}$	
Tumor cells PD-L1	High	Low	Low	Negative effect
Tumor infiltration by TILs	High	Absent	Absent	Positive effect

Stratification factors	Tumor microenvironment subtypes			Cancer immune set point
Antigen immunogenicity	High	Low	Low	Positive effect
KRAS, BRAF, B2M↘ MHC↘	High	Low	Low	Negative effect
IDO				
Hypoxia	High	Low	Low	Negative effect
Tumor microenvironment				
Immune cells	High	High	Very low/absent	
Immune cells phenotypes	Effector cells^{high}	Effector cells^{low}	Very rare myeloid and CD8+ cells	Negative/ positive effect
Spatial relationship	Immunosuppressive cells^{low}	Immunosuppressive cells^{high}		
Immune cells PD-L1	High	Low	Low	Positive effect
Immune gene signatures	High	Low	Low	Positive effect
Fas-L, TGF-β, LOX, VEGF, collagen, fibronectin, CXCL12	Low	High	Low	Negative effect
Host immunity/genetics				
T-cell clonal diversity	High clonality	Low clonality	Low clonality	Negative/ positive effect
Priming of immune response	High	Low	Low	Positive effect
General antibody response	Robust	Weak	Weak	Positive effect
Chronic inflammation/ cytokines	Proinflammatory cytokines	Immunosuppressive cytokines	Immunosuppressive cytokines	Negative/ positive effect
Germline polymorphism: TLR4, TNF-α, NF-κB, NOD2, JAK-STAT, inflammasome pathway	Present	Absent	Absent	Negative effect
Environment				
Gut microbiota				Positive effect
Stress hormones				Negative effect
Glucocorticoids				
Immunotherapy	Sensitivity	Resistance	Resistance	
Therapeutic strategy	Immune checkpoint inhibitors Other immunotherapies	Surgery, radiotherapy chemotherapy, vaccination Adaptive cellular therapy	Surgery, radiotherapy chemotherapy, vaccination Adaptive cellular therapy	

Table 4. A summary table describes the stratification factors implicated in the interactions between immune system, tumor microenvironment, and tumor cells, which can influence immunotherapy and therapeutic strategies (immunophenotype, tumor genome/epigenome, tumor microenvironment, Microbiota, environmental factors, host immunity and genetics). This table proposes global tumor microenvironment morphological-, immunophenotypical- and biological-based subtypes with linked immune biomarkers.

Disclosure-conflict of interest

The authors declare that they have no competing interests.

Author details

Kinan Drak Alsibai[1] and Didier Meseure[2]*

*Address all correspondence to: didier.meseure@curie.fr

1 Department of Anatomic Pathology and Cytology, Raincy-Montfermeil Intercommunal Hospital Group, Montfermeil, France

2 Platform of Experimental Pathology, Curie Institute, Paris, France

References

[1] Stanta G, Jahn SW, Bonin S, Hoefler G. Tumour heterogeneity: Principles and practical consequences. Virchows Archiv. 2016;**469**:371-384

[2] Meseure D, Drak Alsibai K, Nicolas A. Pivotal role of pervasive neoplastic and stromal cells reprogramming in circulating tumor cells dissemination and metastatic colonization. Cancer Microenvironment. 2014;**7**(3):95-115. DOI: 10.1007/s12307-014-0158-2

[3] Drak Alsibai K, Meseure D. Tumor microenvironment and noncoding RNAs as co-drivers of epithelial–mesenchymal transition and cancer metastasis. Developmental Dynamics. 2017. DOI: 10.1002/dvdy.24548

[4] Turley SJ, Cremasco V, Astarita JL. Immunological hallmarks of stromal cells in the tumour microenvironment. Nature Reviews. Immunology. Nov 2015;**15**(11):669-682. DOI: 10.1038/nri3902

[5] Wang M, Zhao J, Zhang L, et al. Role of tumor microenvironment in tumorigenesis. Journal of Cancer. 2017;**8**(5):761-773. DOI: 10.7150/jca.17648

[6] Tjomsland V, Spångeus A, Sandström P, Borch K, Messmer D, Larsson M. Semi mature blood dendritic cells exist in patients with ductal pancreatic adenocarcinoma owing to inflammatory factors released from the tumor. PLoS One. 2010;**5**(10):e13441

[7] Wagner M, Bjerkvig R, Wiig H, Melero-Martin JM, Lin R-Z, Klagsbrun M, Dudley AC. Inflamed tumor-associated adipose tissue is a depot for macrophages that stimulate tumor growth and angiogenesis. Angiogenesis. 2012;**15**(3):481-495. DOI: 10.1007/s10456-012-9276-y

[8] Lee J, Hong BS, Ryu HS, et al. Transition into inflammatory cancer-associated adipocytes in breast cancer microenvironment requires microRNA regulatory mechanism. Ahmad A, editor. PLoS One. 2017;**12**(3):e0174126. DOI: 10.1371/journal.pone.0174126

[9] Navarro R, Compte M, Álvarez-Vallina L, Sanz L. Immune regulation by pericytes: Modulating innate and adaptive immunity. Frontiers in Immunology. 2016;**7**:480. DOI: 10.3389/fimmu.2016.00480

[10] Palm MM, Dallinga MG, van Dijk E, Klaassen I, Schlingemann RO, Merks RMH. Computational screening of tip and stalk cell behavior proposes a role for Apelin signaling in sprout progression. Csikász-Nagy A, editor. PLoS One. 2016;**11**(11):e0159478. DOI: 10.1371/journal.pone.0159478

[11] Ghajar CM, Peinado H, Mori H, et al. The perivascular niche regulates breast tumor dormancy. Nature Cell Biology. 2013;**15**(7):807-817. DOI: 10.1038/ncb2767

[12] Pundavela J, Roselli S, Faulkner S, et al. Nerve fibers infiltrate the tumor microenvironment and are associated with nerve growth factor production and lymph node invasion in breast cancer. Molecular Oncology. 2015;**9**(8):1626-1635. DOI: 10.1016/j.molonc.2015.05.001

[13] Mancino M, Ametller E, Gascón P, Almendro V. The neuronal influence on tumor progression. Biochimica Biophysica Acta. Dec 2011;**1816**(2):105-118. DOI: 10.1016/j.bbcan.2011.04.005

[14] Rosso M, Muñoz M, Berger M. The role of neurokinin-1 receptor in the microenvironment of inflammation and cancer. The Scientific World Journal. 2012;**2012**:381434. DOI: 10.1100/2012/381434

[15] Ullah I, Subbarao RB, Rho GJ. Human mesenchymal stem cells—Current trends and future prospective. Bioscience Reports. 2015;**35**(2):e00191. DOI: 10.1042/BSR20150025

[16] Beckermann BM, Kallifatidis G, Groth A, et al. VEGF expression by mesenchymal stem cells contributes to angiogenesis in pancreatic carcinoma. British Journal of Cancer. 2008;**99**(4):622-631. DOI: 10.1038/sj.bjc.6604508

[17] Guo W, Giancotti FG. Integrin signalling during tumour progression. Nature Reviews. Molecular Cell Biology. 2004;**5**(10):816-826

[18] Parsons JT, Horwitz AR, Schwartz MA. Cell adhesion: Integrating cytoskeletal dynamics and cellular tension. Nature Reviews. Molecular Cell Biology. 2010;**11**(9):633-643. DOI: 10.1038/nrm2957

[19] Hadrup S, Donia M, Thor Straten P. Effector CD4 and CD8 T cells and their role in the tumor microenvironment. Cancer Microenvironment. 2013;**6**(2):123-133

[20] Lanier LL. NKG2D receptor and its ligands in host defense. Cancer Immunology Research. 2015;**3**(6):575-582. DOI: 10.1158/2326-6066.CIR-15-0098

[21] Pandiyan P, Conti HR, Zheng L, Peterson AC, Mathern DR, Hernández-Santos N, Edgerton M, Gaffen SL, Lenardo MJ. $CD4^+$ $CD25^+$ $Foxp3^+$regulatory T cells promote Th17 cells in vitro and enhance host resistance in mouse *Candida albicans* Th17 cell infection model. Immunity. 2011;**34**(3):422-434. DOI: 10.1016/j.immuni.2011.03.002

[22] Lin SC, Chen KH, Lin CH, Kuo CC, Ling QD, Chan CH. The quantitative analysis of peripheral blood FOXP3-expressing T cells in systemic lupus erythematosus and rheumatoid arthritis patients. European Journal of Clinical Investigation. 2007;**37**(12):987-996

[23] Shurin MR, Shurin GV, Lokshin A, Yurkovetsky ZR, Gutkin DW, Chatta G, Zhong H, Han B, Ferris RL. Intratumoral cytokines chemokines growth factors and tumor infiltrating dendritic cells: Friends or enemies? Cancer Metastasis Reviews. 2006;**25**(3):333-356

[24] Steinman RM. Dendritic cells: Understanding immunogenicity. European Journal of Immunology. 2007;**37**(Suppl 1):S53-S60

[25] Colonna M, Trinchieri G, Liu YJ. Plasmacytoid dendritic cells in immunity. Nature Immunology. 2004;**5**(12):1219-1226

[26] Murdoch C, Muthana M, Coffelt SB, Lewis CE. The role of myeloid cells in the promotion of tumour angiogenesis. Nature Reviews. Cancer. 2008;**8**(8):618-631

[27] Qian BZ, Pollard JW. Macrophage diversity enhances tumor progression and metastasis. Cell. 2010;**141**(1):39-51

[28] Mukhtar RA, Nseyo O, Campbell MJ, Esserman LJ. Tumor-associated macrophages in breast cancer as potential biomarkers for new treatments and diagnostics. Expert Review of Molecular Diagnostics. 2011;**11**(1):91-100

[29] Chimal-Ramírez GK, Espinoza-Sánchez NA, Fuentes-Panana EM. Protumor activities of the immune response: Insights in the mechanisms of immunological shift, oncotraining, and oncopromotion. Journal of Oncology. 2013;**2013**:835956. DOI: 10.1155/2013/835956

[30] Goc J, Fridman WH, Sautès-Fridman C, Dieu-Nosjean MC. Characteristics of tertiary lymphoid structures in primary cancers. Oncoimmunology. 2013;**2**(12):e26836

[31] Zhu G, Falahat R, Wang K, Mailloux A, Artzi N, Mulé JJ. Tumor-associated tertiary lymphoid structures: Gene-expression profiling and their bioengineering. Frontiers in Immunology. 2017;**8**:767. DOI: 10.3389/fimmu.2017.00767

[32] Sautès-Fridman C, Lawand M, Giraldo NA, et al. Tertiary lymphoid structures in cancers: Prognostic value, regulation, and manipulation for therapeutic intervention. Frontiers in Immunology. 2016;**7**:407. DOI: 10.3389/fimmu.2016.00407

[33] Paludan S, Bowie A. Immune sensing of DNA. Immunity. 2013;**38**:870-880

[34] Li K, Qu S, Chen X, Wu Q, Shi M. Promising targets for cancer immunotherapy: TLRs, RLRs, and STING-mediated innate immune pathways. International Journal of Molecular Sciences. 2017;**18**. pii: E404. DOI: 10.3390/ijms18020404

[35] Chen DS, Mellman I. Oncology meets immunology: The cancer-immunity cycle. Immunity. 2013;**39**(1):1-10. DOI: 10.1016/j.immuni.2013.07.012

[36] Vasilevko V, Ghochikyan A, Holterman MJ, Agadjanyan MG. CD80 (B7-1) and CD86 (B7-2) are functionally equivalent in the initiation and maintenance of CD4+ T-cell proliferation after activation with suboptimal doses of PHA. DNA and Cell Biology. 2002;**21**(3):137-149

[37] Sharma P, Allison JP. The future of immune checkpoint therapy. Science. 2015;**348**(6230): 56-61. DOI: 10.1126/science.aaa8172

[38] Buchbinder E, Hodi FS, Cytotoxic T. Lymphocyte antigen-4 and immune checkpoint blockade. The Journal of Clinical Investigation. 2015;**125**(9):3377-3383. DOI: 10.1172/JCI80012

[39] Buchbinder EI, Desai A. CTLA-4 and PD-1 pathways: Similarities, differences, and implications of their inhibition. American Journal of Clinical Oncology. 2016;**39**(1):98-106. DOI: 10.1097/COC.0000000000000239

[40] Law AMK, Lim E, Ormandy CJ, Gallego-Ortega D. The innate and adaptive infiltrating immune systems as targets for breast cancer immunotherapy. Endocrine-Related Cancer. 2017;**24**(4):R123-R144. DOI: 10.1530/ERC-16-0404

[41] Gajewski TF. The next hurdle in cancer immunotherapy: Overcoming the non-T cell-inflamed tumor microenvironment. Seminars in Oncology. 2015;**42**(4):663-671. DOI: 10.1053/j.seminoncol.2015.05.011

[42] Ditzel HJ. Human antibodies in cancer and autoimmune disease. Immunologic Research. 2000;**21**(2-3):185-193

[43] Zaenker P, Gray ES, Ziman MR. Autoantibody production in cancer—The humoral immune response toward autologous antigens in cancer patients. Autoimmunity Reviews. 2016;**15**(5):477-483. DOI: 10.1016/j.autrev.2016.01.017

[44] Chen Y, Lan Q, Zheng T, et al. Polymorphisms in JAK/STAT signaling pathway genes and risk of non-Hodgkin lymphoma. Leukemia Research. 2013;**37**(9):1120-1124. DOI: 10.1016/j.leukres.2013.05.003

[45] Kaifu T, Nakamura A. Polymorphisms of immunoglobulin receptors and the effects on clinical outcome in cancer immunotherapy and other immune diseases: A general review. International Immunology. 2017;**29**(7):319-325. DOI: 10.1093/intimm/dxx041

[46] Roy S, Trinchieri G. Microbiota: A key orchestrator of cancer therapy. Nature Reviews Cancer. May 2017;**17**(5):271-285. DOI: 10.1038/nrc.2017.13

[47] Chen DS, Mellman I. Elements of cancer immunity and the cancer-immune set point. Nature. Jan 18, 2017;**541**(7637):321-330. DOI: 10.1038/nature21349

[48] Klintrup K, Mäkinen JM, Kauppila S, Väre PO, Melkko J, Tuominen H, Tuppurainen K, Mäkelä J, Karttunen TJ, Mäkinen MJ. Inflammation and prognosis in colorectal cancer. European Journal of Cancer. Nov 2005;**41**(17):2645-2654

[49] Park JH, Richards CH, McMillan DC, Horgan PG, Roxburgh CS. The relationship between tumour stroma percentage, the tumour microenvironment and survival in patients with primary operable colorectal cancer. Annals of Oncology. 2014;**25**:644-651

[50] Mesker WE, Junggeburt JMC, Szuhai K, et al. The carcinoma–stromal ratio of colon carcinoma is an independent factor for survival compared to lymph node status and tumor stage. Cellular Oncology: The Official Journal of the International Society for Cellular Oncology. 2007;**29**(5):387-398. DOI: 10.1155/2007/175276

[51] Park JH, McMillan DC, Powell AG, Richards CH, Horgan PG, Joanne Edwards J, Roxburgh CS. Evaluation of a tumor microenvironment–based prognostic score in primary operable colorectal cancer. Clinical Cancer Research. 2015;**21**(4):882-888. DOI: 10.1158/1078-0432.CCR-14-1686

[52] Becht E, Giraldo NA, Lacroix L, Buttard B, Elarouci N, Petitprez F, Selves J, Laurent-Puig P, Sautès-Fridman C, Fridman WH, de Reyniès A. Estimating the population abundance of tissue-infiltrating immune and stromal cell populations using gene expression. Genome Biology. Oct 20, 2016;**17**(1):218

[53] Guinney J, Dienstmann R, Wang X, de Reynies A, Schlicker A, Soneson C, et al. The consensus molecular subtypes of colorectal cancer. Nature Medicine. 2015;**21**:1350-1356

[54] Petitprez F, Vano YA, Becht E, Giraldo NA, de Reyniès A, Sautès-Fridman C, Fridman WH. Transcriptomic analysis of the tumor microenvironment to guide prognosis and immunotherapies. Cancer Immunology, Immunotherapy. Sep 7, 2017. DOI: 10.1007/s00262-017-2058-z

[55] Meseure D, Vacher S, Drak Alsibai K, Trassard M, Nicolas A, Leclere R, Lerebours F, Guinebretiere JM, Marangoni E, Lidereau R, Bieche I. Biopathological significance of TLR9 expression in cancer cells and tumor microenvironment across invasive breast carcinomas subtypes. Cancer Microenvironment. 2016;**9**:107-118

[56] Robinson BD, Sica GL, Liu YF, Rohan TE, Gertler FB, Condeelis JS, Jones JG. Tumor microenvironment of metastasis in human breast carcinoma: A potential prognostic marker linked to hematogenous dissemination. Clinical Cancer Research: An Official Journal of the American Association for Cancer Research. 2009;**15**(7):2433-2441. DOI: 10.1158/1078-0432.CCR-08-2179

[57] Rohan TE, Xue X, Lin H-M, et al. Tumor microenvironment of metastasis and risk of distant metastasis of breast cancer. Journal of the National Cancer Institute. 2014;**106**(8): dju136. DOI: 10.1093/jnci/dju136

[58] Salgado R, Denkert C, Demaria S, Sirtaine N, Klauschen F, Pruneri G, Wienert S, Van den Eynden G, Baehner FL, Penault-Llorca F, Perez EA, Thompson EA, Symmans WF, Richardson AL, Brock J, Criscitiello C, Bailey H, Ignatiadis M, Floris G, Sparano J, Kos Z, Nielsen T, Rimm DL, Allison KH, Reis-Filho JS, Loibl S, Sotiriou C, Viale G, Badve S, Adams S, Willard-Gallo K, Loi S. The evaluation of tumor-infiltrating lymphocytes (TILs) in breast cancer: Recommendations by an International TILs Working Group 2014. Annals of Oncology. 2015;**26**(2):259-271

[59] Taube JM, Anders RA, Young GD, Xu H, Sharma R, McMiller TL, et al. Colocalization of inflammatory response with B7-h1 expression in human melanocytic lesions supports an adaptive resistance mechanism of immune escape. Science Translational Medicine. 2012;**4**(127):127ra37

[60] Teng MWL, Ngiow SF, Ribas A, Smyth MJ. Classifying cancers based on T cell infiltration and PD-L1. Cancer Research. 2015;**75**(11):2139-2145. DOI: 10.1158/0008-5472.CAN-15-0255

[61] Herbst RS, Soria JC, Kowanetz M, Fine GD, Hamid O, Gordon MS, et al. Predictive correlates of response to the anti-PD-L1 antibody MPDL3280A in cancer patients. Nature. 2014;**515**(7528):563-567

[62] D'Incecco A, Andreozzi M, Ludovini V, Rossi E, Capodanno A, Landi L, et al. PD-1 and PD-L1 expression in molecularly selected non-small-cell lung cancer patients. British Journal of Cancer. 2015;**112**(1):95-102

[63] Schalper KA, Brown J, Carvajal-Hausdorf D, McLaughlin J, Velcheti V, Syrigos KN, Herbst RS, Rimm DL. Objective measurement and clinical significance of TILs in non-small cell lung cancer. Journal of the National Cancer Institute. 2015;**107**(3):pii:dju435. DOI: 10.1093/jnci/dju435

[64] Gajewski TF, Woo SR, Zha Y, Spaapen R, Zheng Y, Corrales L, Spranger S. Cancer immunotherapy strategies based on overcoming barriers within the tumor microenvironment. Current Opinion in Immunology. Apr 2013;**25**(2):268-276. DOI: 10.1016/j.coi.2013.02.009

[65] Scheel AH, Dietel M, Heukamp LC, Jöhrens K, Kirchner T, Reu S, Rüschoff J, Schildhaus HU, Schirmacher P, Tiemann M, Warth A, Weichert W, Fischer RN, Wolf J, Buettner R. Harmonized PD-L1 immunohistochemistry for pulmonary squamous-cell and adenocarcinomas. Modern Pathology. Oct 2016;**29**(10):1165-1172. DOI: 10.1038/modpathol.2016

[66] Hirsch FR, McElhinny A, Stanforth D, Ranger-Moore J, Jansson M, Kulangara K, Richardson W, Towne P, Hanks D, Vennapusa B, Mistry A, Kalamegham R, Averbuch S, Novotny J, Rubin E, Emancipator K, McCaffery I, Williams JA, Walker J, Longshore J, Tsao MS, Kerr KM. PD-L1 immunohistochemistry assays for lung cancer: Results from phase 1 of the blueprint PD-L1 IHC assay comparison project. Journal of Thoracic Oncology. Feb 2017;**12**(2):208-222. DOI: 10.1016/j.jtho.2016.11.2228

[67] Reck M, Rodríguez-Abreu D, Robinson AG, Hui R, Csőszi T, Fülöp A, Gottfried M, Peled N, Tafreshi A, Cuffe S, O'Brien M, Rao S, Hotta K, Leiby MA, Lubiniecki GM, Shentu Y, Rangwala R, Brahmer JR. KEYNOTE-024 investigators. Pembrolizumab versus chemotherapy for PD-L1-positive non-small-cell lung cancer. The New England Journal of Medicine. Nov 10, 2016;**375**(19):1823-1833

[68] Emens LA, Butterfield LH, Hodi FS, Marincola FM, Kaufman HL. Cancer immunotherapy trials: Leading a paradigm shift in drug development. Journal for Immunotherapy of Cancer. 2016;**4**:42. DOI: 10.1186/s40425-016-0146-9

[69] Harris SJ, Brown J, Lopez J, Yap TA. Immuno-oncology combinations: Raising the tail of the survival curve. Cancer Biology & Medicine. 2016;**13**(2):171-193. DOI: 10.20892/j.issn.2095-3941.2016.0015

[70] Alexander W. The checkpoint immunotherapy revolution: What started as a trickle has become a flood, despite some daunting adverse effects; new drugs, indications, and combinations continue to emerge. Pharmacy and Therapeutics. 2016;**41**(3):185-191

[71] Melero I, Berman DM, Aznar MA, Korman AJ, Pérez Gracia JL, Haanen J. Evolving synergistic combinations of targeted immunotherapies to combat cancer. Nature Reviews Cancer. Aug 2015;**15**(8):457-472. DOI: 10.1038/nrc3973

[72] Pennock GK, Chow LQM. The evolving role of immune checkpoint inhibitors in cancer treatment. The Oncologist. 2015;**20**(7):812-822. DOI: 10.1634/theoncologist.2014-0422

[73] Gibney GT, Weiner LM, Atkins MB. Predictive biomarkers for checkpoint inhibitor-based immunotherapy. The Lancet Oncology. Dec 2016;**17**(12):e542-e551. DOI: 10.1016/S1470-2045(16)30406-5

[74] Yuasa T, Masuda H, Yamamoto S, Numao N, Yonese J. Biomarkers to predict prognosis and response to checkpoint inhibitors. International Journal of Clinical Oncology. 2017;**22**(4):629-634. DOI: 10.1007/s10147-017-1122-1

[75] Masucci GV, Cesano A, Hawtin R, et al. Validation of biomarkers to predict response to immunotherapy in cancer: Vol. I—Pre-analytical and analytical validation. Journal for Immunotherapy of Cancer. 2016;**4**:76. DOI: 10.1186/s40425-016-0178-1

[76] Yuan J, Hegde PS, Clynes R, Foukas PG, Harari A, Kleen TO, Kvistborg P, Maccalli C, Maecker HT, Page DB, Robins H, Song W, Stack EC, Wang E, Whiteside TL, Zhao Y, Zwierzina H, Butterfield LH, Fox BA. Novel technologies and emerging biomarkers for personalized cancer immunotherapy. Journal for Immunotherapy of Cancer. 2016;**4**:3. DOI: 10.1186/s40425-016-0107-3

[77] Stack EC, Wang C, Roman KA, Hoyt CC. Multiplexed immunohistochemistry, imaging, and quantitation: A review, with an assessment of Tyramide signal amplification, multispectral imaging and multiplex analysis. Methods. Nov 2014;**70**(1):46-58. DOI: 10.1016/j.ymeth.2014.08.016

Chapter 3

Histopathology in Zebrafish (*Danio rerio*) to Evaluate the Toxicity of Medicine: An Anti-Inflammatory Phytomedicine with Janaguba Milk (*Himatanthus drasticus* Plumel)

Igor Victor Ferreira dos Santos,
Gisele Custódio de Souza, Giovanna Rocha Santana,
Jonatas Lobato Duarte, Caio Pinho Fernandes,
Hady Keita, Josué Arturo Velázquez-Moyado,
Andrés Navarrete, Irlon Maciel Ferreira,
Helison Oliveira Carvalho and
José Carlos Tavares Carvalho

Additional information is available at the end of the chapter

http://dx.doi.org/10.5772/intechopen.76670

Abstract

The zebrafish Danio rerio appears to be as an alternative experimental model mainly used on toxicological evaluations since the 1990s. In this chapter, we illustrate using a histopathological study the evaluation of a complex phytopreparation with janaguba milk (TPJM, used in popular medicine), which was administrated in zebrafish by immersion in water. We determined (1) lethal concentration 50 (LC_{50}) – 1188.54 μg/mL; (2) the behavioral changes; and (3) the acute administration of TPJM modifications (48 h) at concentrations 500, 750, 1000, and 1500 μg/mL, on the histopathological parameters of the gills, kidneys, and liver. Also the concentrations of 1000 and 1500 μg/mL caused significant damage to the gill tissue and produced a high rate of histological changes in the liver. The kidneys showed greater changes at concentrations of 750, 1000, and 1500 μg/mL. Based on the percentage of TPJM extracts that was only 1.85%, the LC_{50} was calculated as 475 mg/kg; according to traditional indication, only 6 tablespoons/day is consumed; and it is possible to infer that only 0.5 g of active ingredient is ingested by an adult user per day, corresponding to a dose of 7.14 mg/kg, which is far from the toxic effects, demonstrating low toxicity of TPJM.

IntechOpen

Keywords: *Danio rerio, Himatanthus drasticus*, toxicity, histopathology, traditional phytopreparation

1. Introduction

With the increasing pressure for animal welfare, many research groups have been increasingly restricting the use of mammals such as rodents and rabbits in the experimentations. Also, laws, discussions, projects, and committees aimed at reducing the number of animals used in toxicological experiments, forcing a reflection on the subject and the implementation of preliminary tests to draw conclusions that allow the reduction of animal use.

In this context, the zebrafish, *Danio rerio*, appears as an alternative experimental model. This specimen is now used as an experimental model in toxicology since the 1990s [1].

Some studies have demonstrated the importance of these animal species for the development of histopathological studies for the experimentation with new drugs. What has been observed are the relationships between the behavioral profiles within the tissue physiopathology in zebrafish, so it is possible to extrapolate the results to the human tissue changes.

Most of the natural products used in folk medicine do not have scientific backgrounds that prove and elucidate its action mechanism and ensure their use. The toxicological studies of TPJM have not been elucidated in order to measure its possible harm to human health.

Several species of the *Himatanthus* genus have been studied for their chemical composition. Therefore, various chemical classes and several substances of medicinal interest have been isolated and reported in the last years [2]. The metabolites isolated from *Himatanthus* and *Plumeria* species are mainly monoterpene, iridoid-type compounds with the structure of tetrahydrocyclo pentan-pyran [2].

The *H. drasticus* latex has popular knowledge and it is used against lung cancer and lymphatic, intestinal worms, fever, and gastric ulcers [3]. Studies developed by de Mesquita et al. [4] of the *H. drasticus* roots have indicated antiparasitic activity against *Leishmania donovani* promastigotes. Previous studies with the species *Himatanthus* demonstrated pharmacological activity against human epidermoid nasopharyngeal carcinoma [5].

Himatanthus drasticus, like other species of the genus *Himatanthus*, has rarely correlated their biological activity with the phytochemistry. Colares et al. [6] isolated and identified the triterpene lupeol cinnamate from the ethanolic bark extract, which is suggested that this metabolite presents an antitumor activity. Another research developed was the gastroprotective effect of the latex through gastric injury induced by ethanol and indomethacin [6].

Luz et al. [7] performed a phytochemical screening of the bark of *H. drasticus*, identifying alkaloids and tannins. It also presents coumarins with several biological activities, for example, antimicrobial, anti-inflammatory, antiviral, and antioxidant activity, besides the potential antifungal action and the hypocholesterolemic action of the saponins.

http://dx.doi.org/10.5772/intechopen.76670

Other pharmacological studies conducted by de Sousa et al. [8] demonstrated the low toxicity of the crude methanol extract from the leaves of *H. drasticus* and the antitumor activity in experimental sarcoma 180. Mousinho et al. [9] investigated the antitumor effect of *H. drasticus* latex proteins, proving that it can be associated with the immunostimulatory properties. Lucetti et al. [10] studied the possible mechanism of the anti-inflammatory action of lupeol acetate, which probably involves the opioid system, and Colares et al. [6] described the antinociceptive activity evaluated in the writhing test induced by acetic acid.

The zebrafish has been useful for assessing the toxicity of extracts or products of these isolates [11]. In this chapter, we illustrate with a histopathological study the evaluation of a complex phytopreparation with janaguba milk (TPJM, or only janaguba milk, used in popular medicine), which was applied in zebrafish administrated by immersion in water.

2. Materials and methods

The initial project was submitted to the Ethics Committee on Animal Use of the Federal University of Amapá-CEUA-UNIFAP, Macapá, Amapá, Brazil, receiving approval and registration with the n°004/2015 protocol.

2.1. Obtention and yield of traditional phytopreparation with janaguba milk (Himatanthus drasticus): TPJM

The traditional phytopreparation with janaguba milk was purchased from a popular retailer located in the Crato-CE city, and according to the quality control report provided by the company (Number authenticity 0023-2014), the plant species used in the preparation is *Himatanthus drasticus* Plumel.

The yield of the extract of TPJM was estimated by lyophilization and expressed as a percentage. The lyophilized was analyzed by infrared spectrum and high-performance liquid chromatography (HPLC).

The Fourier-transformed infrared spectra (FT-IR) of the lyophilized TPJM were obtained on a Shimadzu spectrometer, FTIR-8400S model, operating in the Fourier transformer. The spectra were obtained in the region from 4000 to 400 cm^{-1} using KBr pellets (solid samples) with a 4.0 resolution and 64 scans.

For the HPLC chromatographic analysis, 3 mg of the lyophilized TPJM was added to 5 ml of hexane, the partition was performed with 5 ml of methanol, and the methanolic fraction was filtered through a membrane with a pore size of 0.45 μm (Millepore®) and analyzed on a HPLC (Shimadzu Corporation) equipped with auto-injector, diode array detector, and was scanned from 190 to 500 nm. Chromatographic conditions: chromatograms were obtained at 280 nm, the temperature was maintained at 30°C, a reverse phase column was used, Shim-pack VP-ODS (150 × 4.6 mm; 5 μm), and the injection volume was 10 μL using a mixture of the phase A containing acidified water (24%) with acetic acid and methanol (70:30, v/v) and phase B containing acetonitrile, in an isocratic system of proportions 70:30 (v/v) with a flow rate of 1 ml/min. The identification of the peak corresponding to gallic acid was performed in comparison with the standard substance.

2.2. Acute toxicity tests

2.2.1. Experimental animals

Authenticated *D. rerio* species were purchased from the company Acqua New Aquariums and Fish located in Itaguassu-PE, Brazil, under the authorization of the Protocol 526140011289802 (May 7, 2014), registered at IBAMA with No. 82957. The animals were kept in quarantine in a zebrafish platform on the Drug research laboratory (Laboratório de Pesquisa em Fármacos), UNIFAP, Brazil, until the experiments were made.

2.2.2. Assessment of the behavioral parameters of D. rerio under treatment with TPJM

For this study, a total of 90 animals were used, only adults who were 6–8 months were selected for the study. The animals were maintained at a temperature of 26 ± 2°C with a light:dark cycle of 10:14 h. Also we used standardized water for the maintenance of adult fish.

Adult fish were fed with commercial brine shrimp (*Artemia salina*). The animals were treated according to the guide for the care and use of experimental animals. The fish behavior was assessed by a human observer and filmed after 0, 3, 6, 12, 24, 27, 30, and 48 h.

2.2.3. Determination of LC_{50}

Concentrations of 500, 750, 1000, and 1500 μg/mL of the TPJM were tested in order to obtain the median lethal concentration (LC_{50}). Each concentration was performed by triplicate, using 15 animals per assay. The exposition time with the different solutions was 48 h.

2.2.4. Assessment of behavioral parameters

Animals were exposed to the concentrations of 500, 750, 1000, and 1500 μg/mL of the TPJM on a single tank for 48 h, all experiments were done by triplicate (n = 15), tank water was used as a control test. The behavior was assessed by a human observer and filmed after 0, 3, 6, 12, 24, 27, 30, and 48 h of exposure to TPJM. All the responses were characterized at three stages following the protocol previously described by Ribeiro [12].

2.2.5. Monitoring of mortality

Mortality was monitored continuously, and the fish were considered dead when the movement of the operculum and response to mechanical stimulation could no longer be detected. After the experiment, the remaining fish were euthanized by anesthesia by cooling, in agreement with the recommendation of the American Veterinary Medical Association Guidelines for the Euthanasia of Animals (2013 Edition Members).

2.2.6. Evaluation of the histopathological parameters

For the histopathology analysis, the organs (gills, liver, and kidney) were fixed in Bouin solution for 24 h according to the method described by Souza [13]. The analysis of slides was performed under an optical microscope Olympus BX41-Micronal and photographed with MDCE-5C USB 2.0 camera (digital) and by a scanning electron microscopy (microscope Hitachi TM3030PLUS).

2.2.6.1. Measurement of histopathological alterations

We considered some histopathological changes in the gills, liver, and kidneys. The damage was categorized using a semi quantitative analysis, and calculating the average medium assessment (VMA as previously described by Shwaiger [14]), calculated from semi quantitative analysis based on a scale of severity and occurrence of the lesions.

We also used the changes histological index (CHI) described by Poleksic and Mitrovic-Tutundzic [15]. This ratio was based on the branchial lesions, each type of injury being rated as the severity in stages I, II, and III.

Thus, the indices were calculated according to the following equation:

$$\frac{I = \sum_{i-1}^{na} ai + 10 \sum_{i-1}^{nb} bi + 102 \sum_{i-1}^{nc} ci}{N} \quad (1)$$

where: *a*: changes first stage; *b*: changes second stage; *c*: changes third stage; *na*: number of amendments considered to be the first stage; *nb*: number of modifications considered to be second-stage; *nc*: number of amendments considered to be the third stage; *N*: number of analyzed fish per treatment.

In this study, this equation was used to calculate the changing index not only in the gills but also liver and kidney [15]. In the present study, these relationships were extrapolated to the kidneys and the liver. The parameters considered in this chapter are established in **Table 1**.

2.3. Statistical analysis

The LC_{50} values over their 95% confidence intervals were calculated by probit analysis using GraphPad Prism Software Version 5.0. To analyze the histopathological findings a one-way

Values	Effects
0–10	Normal organ functionality
11–20	Organ with mild to moderate changes
21–50	Organ with moderate to severe changes
>100	Organ with irreversible damage

Table 1. Different stages in the histopathological changes seen in the zebrafish.

analysis of variance (ANOVA) followed by the Tukey-Kramer *post-hoc* test were conducted. Data were expressed as the mean ± SEM. Results with $*p < 0.05$, $**p < 0.01$ and $***p < 0.001$ were considered statistically significant.

3. Results

The yield of the extracts of the TPJM obtained by lyophilization was 1.85%. The phytopreparation is composed of diluted exuding latex of janaguba (1:10). This concentration is similar as many of the products marketed commonly used on the folk medicine.

According to FT-IR analysis of the lyophilized TPJM, it is possible to observe an intense broadband of 3414.15 cm^{-1} suggesting the presence of fatty acids in the resin of *Himatanthus drasticus*. Note that the presence of aliphatic carbons in 2852.84 and 2924.21 cm^{-1} is characteristic of the carbon chains of terpenes (**Figure 1**). Lupeol triterpene class can be observed by characteristically the signals 1454.39 and 1377.23 cm^{-1} for the rings; the signal at 1695 cm^{-1} belongs of the stretching of carbon-carbon bond, suggesting the presence of compounds of the triterpene lupeol class [6].

The chromatogram obtained by HPLC of the methanolic fraction of the lyophilized TPJM contains several signals, the peak corresponding to gallic acid showed a retention time of 7.240 min (**Figures 2** and **3**), corroborating the study by Luz et al. [7] which identifies the presence of various classes of phenolic compounds.

The exposure by immersion of *D. rerio* to different concentrations of TPJM triggered significant behavioral changes in the fish only at higher concentrations (1000 and 1500 μg/mL). Such changes were classified into three stages: I, II, and III (**Table 2**).

The behavior of the fish was filmed for 2 min during the intervals of observation. The toxic action of TPJM depends on the concentration administered; at the two lower concentrations, the fish expressed only milder and less changes, whereas, at higher concentrations, severe behavioral changes were observed (**Table 2**).

Table 3 shows the percentage of dead animals by different concentrations of TPJM. These results demonstrate the susceptibility of *D. rerio* to the TPJM in preliminary testing concentrations, although between 20 and 100 μg/mL, no deaths were observed and neither at the concentrations of 500 and 750 μg/mL. The estimated LC_{50} value was calculated as 1188.54 μg/mL (**Figure 4**).

The changes in gill tissue of *D. rerio* by immersion exposure of TPJM are quantified in **Table 4**. Stage I of histopathological changes such as hypertrophy of the respiratory epithelium (composed of the lamellae) and hyperplasia of epithelial cells was present in all the concentrations (**Figure 5**).

The fusion of secondary lamellae was present in all tested concentrations and was more frequent the higher concentrations of 750, 1000, and 1500 μg/mL. Additionally, the complete

http://dx.doi.org/10.5772/intechopen.76670

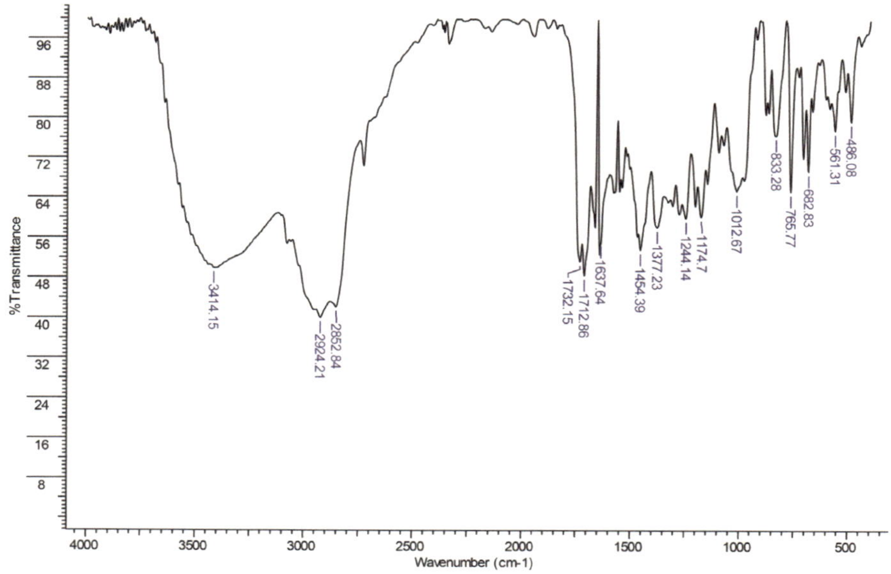

Figure 1. Infrared spectrum, corresponding to the lyophilized TPJM, an intense broadband 3414.15 cm^{-1} suggest the presence of fatty acids in the TPJM. Presence of aliphatic carbons in 2852.84 and 2924.21 cm^{-1} abundant in carbon chains of terpenes.

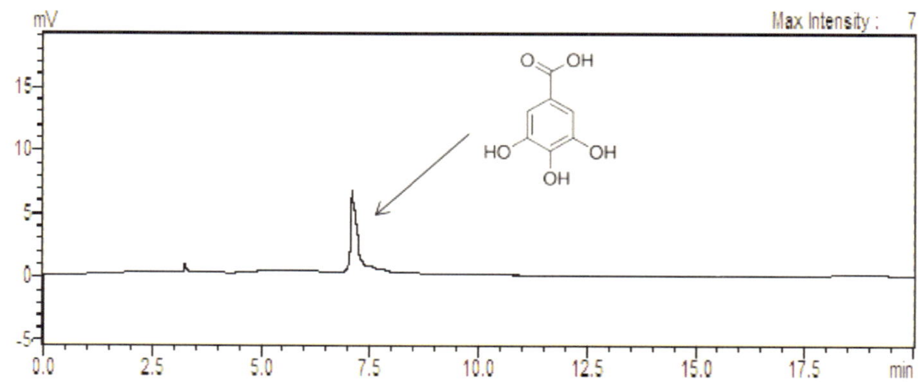

Figure 2. Chromatographic obtained of the gallic acid standard reference with retention peak in 7.240 min.

fusion of all the secondary lamellae is visible only in the higher concentrations of TPJM (**Figure 5**).

The changes in blood vessel lamellar, stage I, were common at all concentrations (**Table 4**). The rupture of blood vessels and subsequent hemorrhage were observed in every treatment. The presence of a lamellar aneurysm in only one concentration was observed (1000 μg/mL of TPJM) (**Figure 5**). These changes are rarely observed in normal conditions. Although the infiltration of

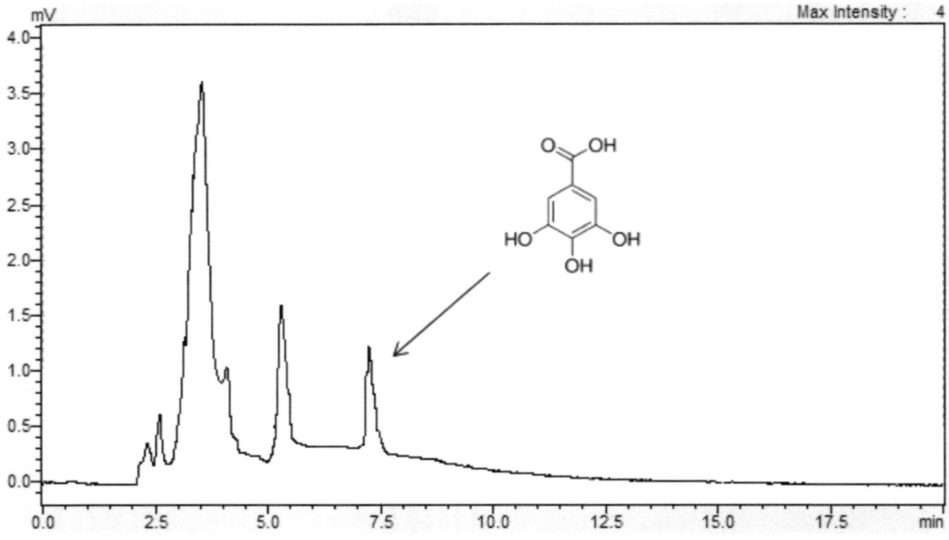

Figure 3. Chromatographic profile of the methanolic fraction from the lyophilized TPJM, with retention peak in 7.240 min equivalent to gallic acid.

		500 μg/mL of TPJM	750 μg/mL of TPJM	1000 μg/mL of TPJM	1500 μg/mL of TPJM	Control
Stage I	0′	1	1	1	1 and 3	
Stage II	0′		1	1 and 2	1 and 2	
Stage III	0′				2 and 3	
Stage I	3 h			1	2	
Stage II	3 h			1	1 and 2	
Stage	3 h			2 and 3	2 and 3	
Stage I	9 h			1		
Stage II	9 h					
Stage III	9 h		2		2	
Stage I	24 h			1		
Stage II	24 h					
Stage III	24 h			2 and 3	2 and 3	
Stage I	27 h			1		
Stage II	27 h					
Stage III	27 h				2	
Stage I	33 h			1		
Stage II	33 h					
Stage III	33 h				2	
Estágio I	48 h			1		
Estágio II	48 h					
Estágio III	48 h				2	

Stage I: (1) increase swimming activity, (2) tail tremors; stage II: (1) circular swimming movement, (2) loss of posture; stage III: (1) loss of motility; (2) animal deposition in the base of the beaker, (3) death.

Table 2. Effects of the concentrations of TPJM on *D. rerio* behaviors in different hours of observations.

http://dx.doi.org/10.5772/intechopen.76670

Concentration of TPJM	500 μg/mL	750 μg/mL	1000 μg/mL	1500 μg/mL	Control
Number of animals death	0	0	4	13	0
Percentagen (%)	0	0	26.7	86.6	0

Table 3. Percentage of animal death with the concentrations of TPJM on ***D. rerio***.

leukocytes in the lamellar epithelium was also not diagnosed, it may lead to aneurysm or even hemorrhage epithelial disruption [16].

In stage III, the necrotic alteration on the *D. rerio* specimens was manifested in the groups treated with 1000 and 1500 μg/mL causing the death of the animals. Cellular degeneration was presented only at the concentrations higher than 750 μg/mL (**Figure 5**).

The quantitative results (**Table 4**) and qualitative results (**Figure 5**) indicate that the exposition caused changes on the gills of *D. rerio*, compared to the control. Furthermore, it is possible to note that concentrations of 1000 and 1500 μg/mL were responsible for the higher IAH (**Figure 6** and **Table 5**).

According to the gills, IAH even with stage III changes such as necrosis can also be classified as functionally organs. **Table 5** shows that the gills are functionally normal in all treatments with TPJM.

The *D. rerio* livers showed histopathological changes in hepatocytes, blood vessels, and bile canaliculi. The *D. rerio* hepatocytes have typical aspects described as in most vertebrates. In **Table 6**, we quantified the occurrence of liver abnormalities in the fish exposed to different concentrations of TPJM. Also, qualitative data show changes in **Figures 7** and **8**. All of the stage I alterations were present in the various treatment concentrations. It may be noted in

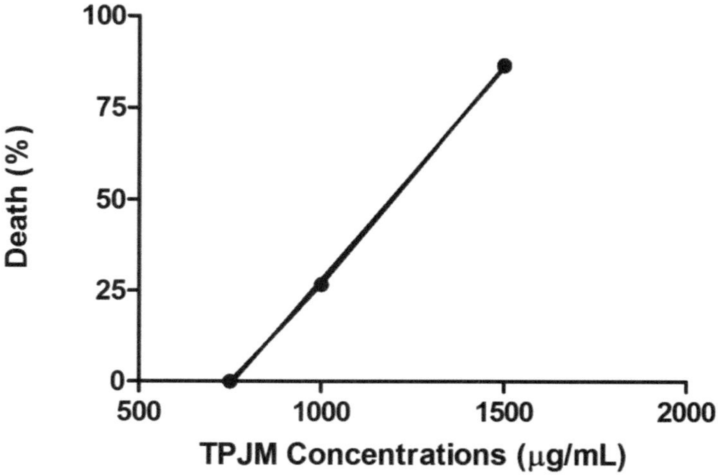

Figure 4. Effects of administration of different TPJM concentrations (500, 750, 1000, 1500 μg/mL) on D. rerio n = 15/group, LC50 = 1188.54 μg/mL.

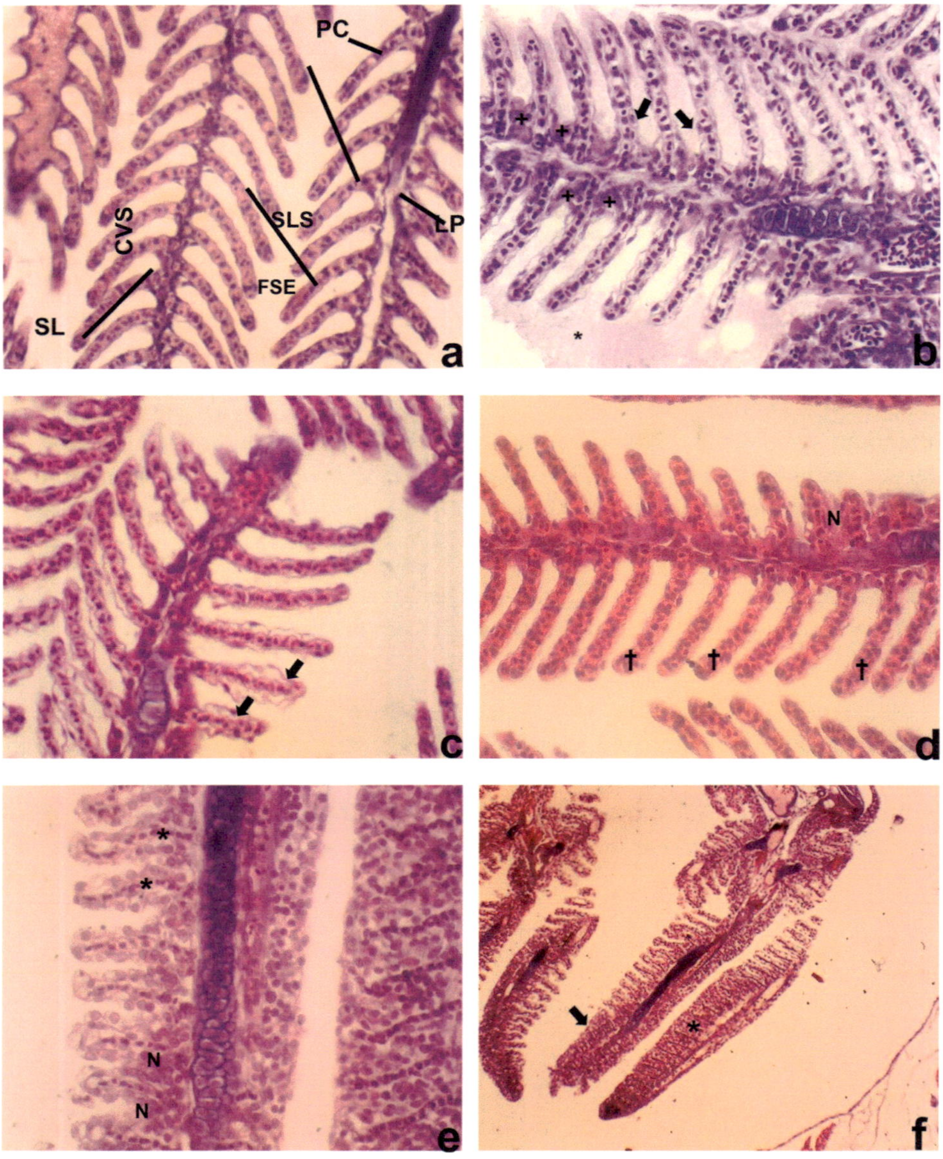

Figure 5. Histopathological changes in the gills of *D. rerio* exposed to different concentrations of TPJM. (a) Normal gill filament on longitudinal histological section. PC—pillar cells; FSE—filament stratified epithelium; SLS—secondary lamellar squamous epithelium; SL—secondary lamellae; CVS—central venous sinus (400×); (b) gill filament on longitudinal histological section exposed to 500 μg/mL of TPJM. Hyperplasia of epithelial cells in the secondary lamellae (+), presence of chloride (black arrow) and mucus secretion (*) (400×). (c) Gill filament on longitudinal histological sections exposed to 750 μg/mL. Epithelial Detachment (black arrow) (400×). (d) Gill filament on longitudinal histological section exposed to concentration of 1000 μg/mL. Vascular congestion, dilation of capillaries (†) and necrosis of respiratory epithelial cells (N). (e) Gill filament on longitudinal histological section exposed to 1500 μg/mL of TPJM. Necrosis of respiratory epithelial cells (N) and capillary derangements (*) (400×). (f) Gill filament on longitudinal histological section exposed to 1500 μg/mL. Fusion of some secondary lamellae (black arrow) and fusion of all secondary lamellae (*) (100×).

Alterations	Stage	Control	500 μg/mL of TPJM	750 μg/mL of TPJM	1000 μg/mL of TPJM	1500 μg/mL of TPJM
HTEC	I	0	86.6	100	100	100
TEpi	I	0	0	0	0	0
DEC(LS)	I	0	86.6	100	100	100
HECBSL	I	0	100	100	100	100
HECSL	I	0	93.3	100	100	100
FPLS	I	0	40	66.6	66.6	100
LeuELS	I	0	0	0	0	0
HP/HTCM	I	0	60	66.6	60	93.3
HP/HTCC	I	0	13.3	93.3	60	100
CCSL	I	0	86.6	93.3	86.6	93.3
MuLS	I	0	26.6	26.6	20	93.3
DiC	I	0	100	100	93.3	100
CDe	I	0	66.6	100	93.3	100
VC	I	0	100	100	93.3	100
Par	I	0	0	0	0	0
CFSSL	I	0	26.6	60.3	60.3	100
CFALSL	II	0	0	0	0	53.3
CD	II	0	0	66.6	73.3	100
ER	II	0	0	0	66.6	100
Hem	II	0	0	0	0	0
An	II	0	0	0	20	0
Fib	III	0	0	0	0	0
Nec	III	0	0	0	66.6	86.7

Each value represents, in percentage, number of damage fishes in relation to total fishes (N = 15) for each concentration. HTEC = hypertrophy of epithelial cells; TEpi = thinning of epithelium; DELC(LS) = displacement or lifting up of epithelial cells (LS); HECBSL: hyperplasia of epithelial cells at the basis of secondary lamellae; HECSL = hyperplasia of epithelial cells on secondary lamellae; LeuELS = presence of leukocytes; HP/HTCM = hyperplasia/hypertrophy of mucous cells; HP/HTCC = hyperplasia/hypertrophy of chloride cells; CCSL = presence of chloride cells on secondary lamellae; MuLS = presence of mucous cells on secondary lamellae; DiC = dilatation of capillaries; CDe = capillary disarrangement; VC = vascular congestion; Par = presence of parasites; CFSSL = complete fusion of some secondary lamellar; CFASL = complete fusion of all secondary lamellae; CD = cellular degeneration: ER = epithelial rupture; Hem = hemorrhage; An = aneurism; Fib = fibrosis; Nec = necrosis.

Table 4. Occurrence of alterations in percentage on gills of treated groups exposed to different concentrations of TPJM.

particular the disruption of hepatic cords, loss or atypical contour of hepatocytes, intense vacuolation, and decreased glycogen amount.

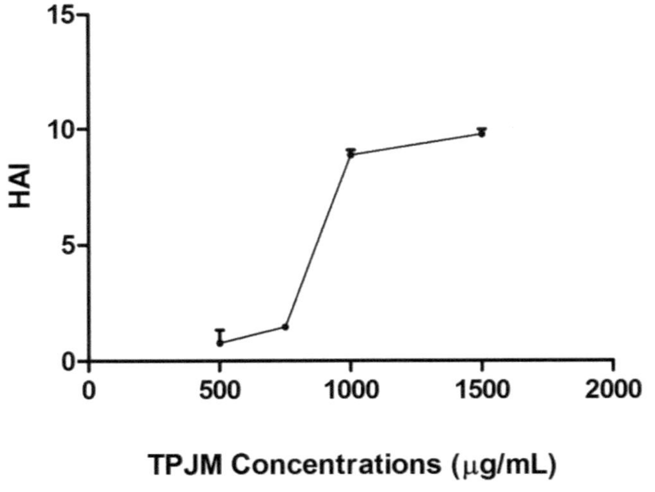

Figure 6. .Mean HAI obtained from histopathological alterations observed on *D. rerio* gills exposed to TPJM (500, 750, 100 and 1500 μg/mL). Each point represents mean ± SEM (N = 15/group). ANOVA followed by Tukey-Kramer test: 500 μg vs. control $p < 0.05$; 750 μg/mL vs. control $p < 0.001$; 1000 vs. control $p < 0.001$; 1500 vs. control $p < 0.001$.

The increase in cell volume of hepatocytes is observed with treatment with TPJM and reflects the hyperfunctional condition of the liver (**Figures 7** and **8**). The increase in hepatic metabolism may also lead to necrosis whereas the core becomes hypertrophic or even degenerates (histopathologic change stage III); both changes are found in the three higher concentrations.

The biliary stagnation was another stage of manifestation I (**Table 6**) observed in treatments with TPJM at all concentrations. However, cholestasis was seen on the 750, 1000, and 1500 μg/mL treatments; it is characterized by a manifestation of a pathophysiological condition (**Figures 7** and **8**) assigned to metabolic failure or the excretion of bile pigments, because the metabolites excreted as bilirubin need to be solubilized in water, a process which occurs only through conjugation with glucuronic acid.

Triplicate	Control	500 μg/mL of TPJM	750 μg/mL of TPJM	1000 μg/mL of TPJM	1500 μg/mL of TPJM
01	0.0	0.80	1.46	9.46	9.53
02	0.0	0.86	1.46	8.8	10.2
03	0.0	0.67	1.46	8.87	9.53
Mean	0.0	0.77	1.46	9.04	9.75
Average standard error	±0.0	±0.56	±0.0	±0.21	±0.22

Table 5. Mean of histological alteration index (HAI) of ***D. rerio*** gills after exposure do different concentrations of TPJM in triplicate (n = 15 animals/group).

Alterations	Stage	Control	500 μg/mL of TPJM	750 μg/mL of TPJM	1000 μg/mL of TPJM	1500 μg/mL of TPJM
HCD	I	0	93.3	100	100	100
OCLA	I	0	100	100	100	100
ONLA	I	0	100	80	100	100
ICV	I	0	100	100	93.3	100
INV	I	0	60	73.4	80	100
CV	I	0	66.7	60	80	100
DRFN	I	0	93.3	100	80	100
IRFBV	I	0	53.4	80	80	100
IRVBV	I	0	20	20	46.7	100
GR	I	0	80	53.4	80	100
BS	II	0	46.7	86.7	93.3	100
Hyp	II	0	6.7	66.7	100	100
DBV	II	0	60	86.7	93.3	100
DBC	II	0	26.7	73.4	93.3	100
NV	II	0	0	66.7	60	100
CD	II	0	0	6.7	20	40
ND	II	0	0	0	26.7	66.7
NA	III	0	0	6.7	0	20
CDis	III	0	0	33.5	80	80

Each value represents, in percentage, number of damage fishes in relation to total fishes (N = 15) for each concentration. HCD = hepatic cordon disarrangement; OCLA = outline cell loss or atypia; ONLA = outline nuclear loss or atypia; ICV = increase in cell volume; INV = increase in nuclear volume; CV = cytoplasmic vacuolation; DRFN = decrease in relative frequency of nuclei; IRFBV = increase in the relative frequency of blood vessels; IRVBV = increase on relative volume of blood vessels; GR = glycogen reduction; BS = biliary stagnation; Hyp = hyperemia; DBV = disruption of blood vessels; DBC = degeneration bile canaliculi; NV = nuclear vacuolation; CD = cytoplasmic degeneration; ND = nuclear degeneration; NA = nuclear atrophy; CDis = cellular disruption.

Table 6. Occurrence of alterations in percentage on liver of treated groups exposed to different concentrations of TPMJ.

The most frequent stage II changes (**Table 6**) were hyperemia, degeneration, and vacuolization (nuclear/cytoplasmic). The redness may indicate an adaptation process which leads to an increased blood flow to the liver tissue, facilitating the transport of macrophages to the damaged tissue and also the growth of the oxygenation of these areas or may indicate a secondary mechanism of detoxification. Changes such as nuclear and cell degeneration and cell strain may indicate contour dysfunctions induced by a toxic agent, since metabolically active areas of the liver are reduced, leading to a possible reduction in the overall functions performed by this organ.

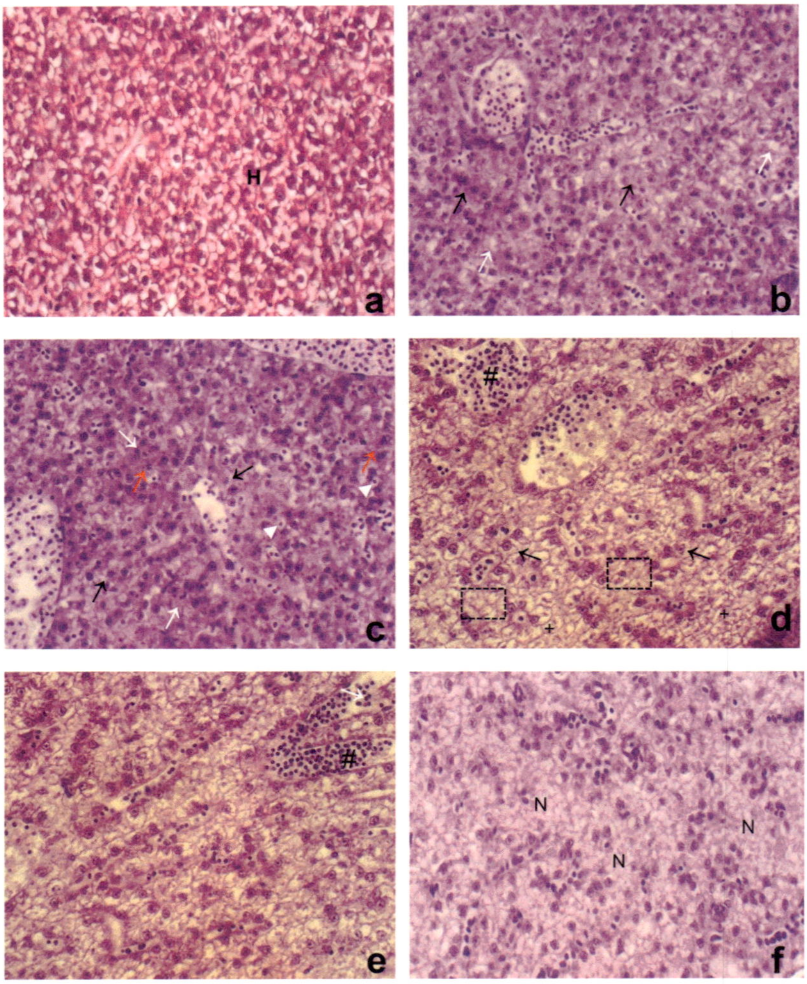

Figure 7. Histopathological changes in the livers of *D. rerio* exposed to different concentrations of TPJM. (a) Normal liver on longitudinal histological section. Hepatocytes (H) (400×). (b) Liver on longitudinal histological section exposed to 500 μg/mL of TPJM. Outline cell atypia (black arrows) and derangement of the hepatic cords (white arrows) (400×). (c) Liver on longitudinal histological section exposed to 750 μg/mL of TPJM. Nuclear atrophy (black arrows), cytoplasmic degeneration (white arrows), biliary stagnation (white arrow heads) and nuclear degeneration (red arrows) (400×). (d) Liver on longitudinal histological section exposed to 1000 μg/mL of TJPM. Glycogen reduction (+), decrease in the relative frequency of nuclei (dotted area), nuclear vacuolation (black arrows) and hyperemia (#). (e) Liver on longitudinal histological section exposed to 1500 μg/mL of TPJM. Hyperemia (#) and vessel rupture (white arrow) (400×). (f) Liver on longitudinal section exposed to 1500 μg/mL of TJPM. Focal necrosis (N) (400×).

As for stage III changes (**Table 6**), these were noted in the three major concentrations and are represented by the rupture vessels and overall or focal necrosis.

Table 6 and **Figures 7** and **8** show that the concentrations of TPJM (750, 1000, and 1500 μg/mL) caused significant changes when compared to the control; also no alterations were observed

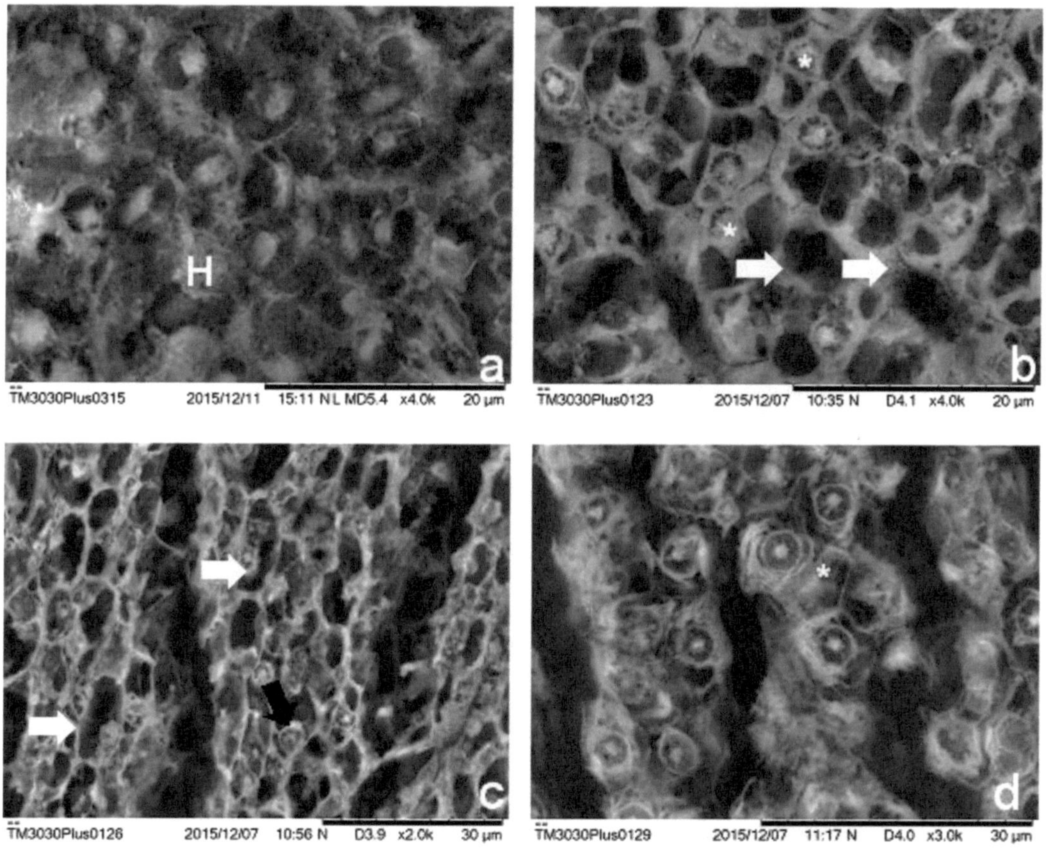

Figure 8. Histopathological analysis by scanning electron microscopy of the livers of *D. rerio* exposed to different concentrations of TPJM. (a) Normal liver on longitudinal histological section. Hepatocytes (H) (3000×). (b) Liver on longitudinal histological section exposed to 750 μg/mL of TPJM. Outline cell atypia (*), nuclear atypia (white arrow) (4000×). (c) Liver on longitudinal histological section exposed to 1000 μg/mL of TJPM. Outline cell atypia (white arrow), nuclear vacuolation (black arrow) (2000×). (d) Liver on longitudinal histological section exposed to 1500 μg/mL of TPJM. Nuclear degeneration (*) (3000×).

at 500 μg/mL. Interestingly, when comparing the IAH liver with the ones exposed with TPJM, it is also possible to observe that only the comparison between the concentrations of 750 versus 1000 μg/mL was not significant (**Table 7**).

The pathological changes in the kidneys of *Danio rerio* were evaluated in the lymphoid tissue, glomeruli, and renal tubules and blood vessels. **Table 8** shows the quantitation of kidney histopathological changes and **Figures 7** and **8** show changes in the qualitative data. Thus, virtually all stage I changes were observed in the various treatment concentrations.

Necrosis was ranked in this study as change stage III, being observed at the three highest exposure concentrations of TPJM (**Table 8**).

Triplicate	Control	500 µg/mL of TPJM	750 µg/mL of TPJM	1000 µg/mL of TPJM	1500 µg/mL of TPJM
01	0.0	1.2	10.7	11.3	18.7
02	0.0	2.7	10.7	12	12
03	0.0	3.9	11.3	10.7	18.7
Mean	0.0	2.6	10.9	11.3	16.5
Average standard error	±0.0	±0.78	±0.2	±0.38	±2.23

Table 7. Mean of histological alteration index (HAI) of ***D. rerio*** liver after exposure do different concentrations of TPJM in triplicate (n = 15 animals/group).

Alterations	Stage	Control	500 µg/mL of TPJM	750 µg/mL of TPJM	1000 µg/mL of TPJM	1500 µg/mL of TPJM
LCO	I	0	60	80	100	100
LDH	I	0	93.3	100	100	100
HTC	I	0	93.3	93.3	100	100
TDis	I	0	93.3	100	100	100
GDis	I	0	93.3	86.7	93.3	100
IBCS	I	0	80	46.7	33.3	20
DBCS	I	0	26.6	73.3	60	93.3
DGC	I	0	20	53.3	26.6	33.3
PRT	I	0	20	13.3	0	40
DRFG	I	0	46.7	60	80	86.7
DilBV	I	0	60	93.3	73.3	100
ITL	I	0	60	46.7	46.7	66.7
TO	I	0	100	73.3	93.3	100
SDTH	II	0	13.3	73.3	80	100
TD	II	0	86.7	93.3	100	100
GD	II	0	33.3	20	93.3	100
CDTC	II	0	86.7	73.3	100	100
NDTC	II	0	33.3	60	100	100
PLTBC	II	0	53.3	60	13.3	100
Hyp	II	0	6.7	73.3	93.3	100
RBV	III	0	0	0	0	40
Nec	III	0	0	53.3	66.7	100

Each value represents, in percentage, number of damage fishes in relation to total fishes (N = 15) for each concentration. LCO = loss of cellular outline or atypical cellular outline on lymphoid tissue; LDH = low degeneration of hyaline; HTC = hypertrophy of tubular cells; TDis = tubular disorganization; GDis = glomerular disorganization; IBCS = increase on Bowman´s capsule space; DBCS = decrease on Bowman´s capsule space; DGC = dilatation of glomerular capillaries; PRT = presence of regenerated tubules or "new" nephrons; PSG = presence of several granules PAS positive on tubular cells; DRFG = decrease in the relative frequency of glomerulus; DilBV = dilatation of blood vessels; ITL = increase in tubular lumen; TO = tubular obstruction; SDTH = severe degeneration on tubular hyaline; TD = tubular degeneration; GD = glomerular degeneration; CDTC = cytoplasmic degeneration of tubular cells; NDTC = nuclear degeneration of tubular cells; PLTBC = presence of lymphoid tissue on Bowman´s capsule; Hyp = hyperemia; RBV = rupture of blood vessels; Nec = necrosis.

Table 8. Occurrence of alterations in percentage on kidney of treated groups exposed to different concentrations of TPMJ.

http://dx.doi.org/10.5772/intechopen.76670

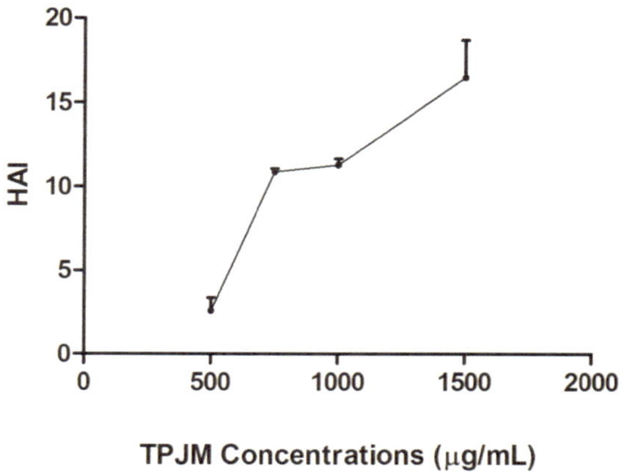

Figure 9. Mean HAI obtained from histopathological alterations observed in liver *D. rerio* exposed to TPJM concentrations (500, 750, 1000 and 1500 μg/mL). Each point represents mean ± SEM (N = 15/group). ANOVA followed by Tukey-Kramer: 500 μg vs. control no significative; 750 μg/mL vs. control $p < 0.001$; 1000 vs. control $p < 0.001$; 1500 vs. control $p < 0.001$.

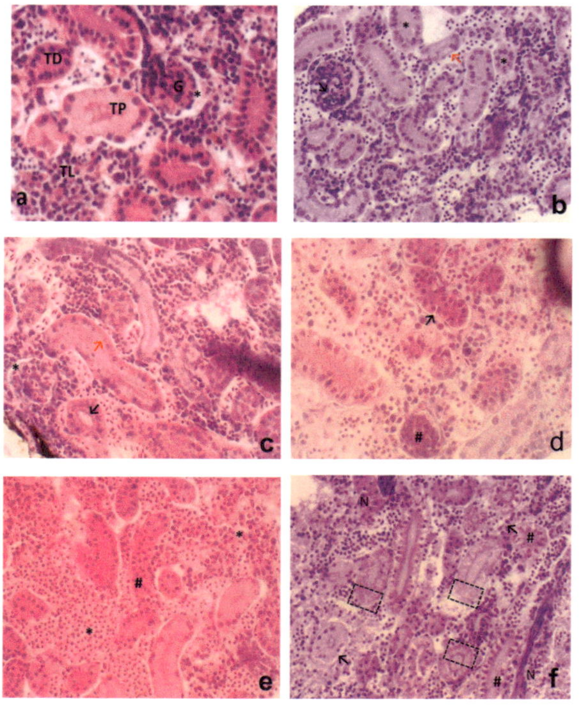

Figure 10. Histopathological changes in the kidney of *D. rerio* exposed to different concentrations of TPJM. (a) Normal kidney on longitudinal histological section. Glomerulus (G). Intercapsular space (*). Lymphoid tissue (TL), distal tubule (TD), proximal tubule (TP). (b) Kidney on longitudinal section exposed to 500 μg/mL of TPJM. Dilated glomerular capillaries (black arrow), tubular obstruction (*) and tubular disorganization (red arrow) (400×). (c) Kidney on longitudinal section exposed to 750 μg/mL of TPJM (400×). Decrease on Bowman's capsule space (*), increase in tubular lumen (black arrow), cytoplasmic degeneration (red arrow). (d) Kidney on longitudinal section exposed to 1000 μg/mL of TPJM (400×). Glomerular degeneration (#) and degeneration of tubular hyaline (black arrow). (e) Kidney on longitudinal section exposed to 1000 μg/mL of TPJM (400×). Tubular degeneration (#) and hyperemia (*). (f) Kidney on longitudinal section exposed to 1500 μg/mL of TPJM. Nuclear degeneration (dotted area), tubular degeneration (#), necrosis (N) and degeneration of tubular hyaline (black arrow).

These histopathological changes were noted at all concentrations of TPJM treatment in an increasing manner about the percentage of occurrence, while the other histopathological changes related to Bowman's capsule (AECB) were not manifested (**Figures 10** and **11**).

The appearance of blood cells, blood cell aggregates, or foreign matter in Bowman's space can also occur [17, 18]. Sometimes the excess of red blood cells in the capillary can lead to the rupture of these vessels and, in this case, it is common to find cells in Bowman's space. Rupture of the capillaries due to the excess of erythrocytes has been observed at the concentration of 1500 μg/mL and it is classified as a stage III change (**Table 9**).

All of these observations can be explained by the phytochemical composition of *H. drasticus*, which has phytochemical markers such as plumeride and isoplumeride, which are typically lipophilic compounds.

The concentrations that caused mortality showed kidneys with mild-to-moderate changes. The concentration of 750 μg/mL has caused changes in this level, demonstrating that there is already kidney damage at this concentration (**Figure 12**).

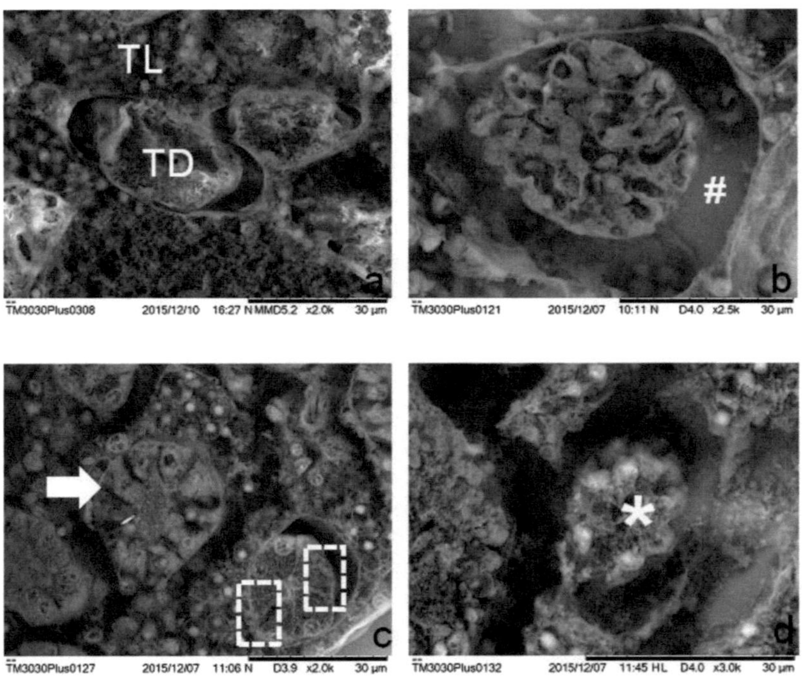

Figure 11. Histopathological analysis by scanning electron microscopy of the kidney of *D. rerio* exposed to different concentrations of TPJM. (a) Normal kidney on longitudinal histological section. Lymphoid tissue (TL) and distal tubule (TD) (2000×). (b) Kidney on longitudinal section exposed to 750 μg/mL of TPJM. Increase on Bowman's capsule space (#) (2500×). (c) Kidney on longitudinal section exposed to 1000 μg/mL of TPJM. Degeneration of tubular hyaline (arrow), nuclear degeneration of tubular cells (dotted area) (2000×). (d) Kidney on longitudinal section exposed to 1500 μg/mL of TPJM. Glomerular degeneration (*) (3000×).

Triplicate	Control	500 μg/mL of TPJM	750 μg/mL of TPJM	1000 μg/mL of TPJM	1500 μg/mL of TPJM
01	0.0	2.73	11.53	12.2	18.67
02	0.0	3.4	12.06	11.33	18.86
03	0.0	4.2	11.53	11.53	18.67
Mean	0.0	3.44	11.70	11.68	18.73
Average standard error	±0.0	±0.42	±0.17	±0.26	±0.06

Table 9. Mean of histological alteration index (HAI) of ***D. rerio*** kidney after exposure do different concentrations of TPJM in triplicate (n = 15 animals/group).

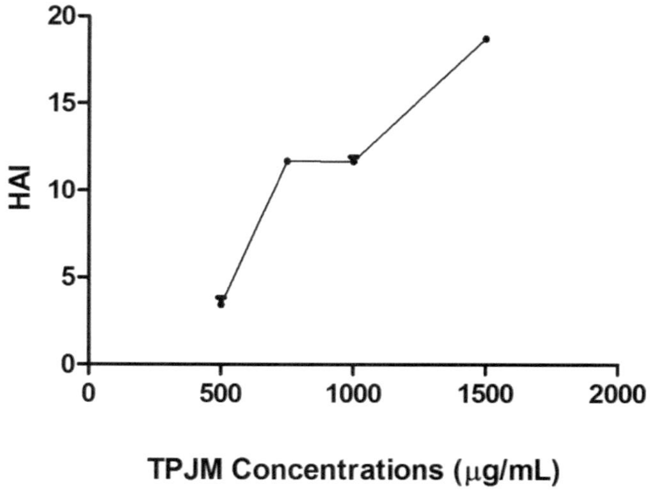

Figure 12. Mean HAI obtained from histopathological alterations observed on *D. rerio* kidneys exposed to TPJM (500, 750, 1000 and 1500 μg/mL). Each point represents the mean ± SEM (N = 15/group). ANOVA followed by Tukey-Kramer test: 500 μg/mL vs. control $p < 0.001$; 750 μg/mL $p < 0.001$; 1000 μg/mL vs. control $p < 0.001$; 1500 μg/mL vs. control $p < 0.001$.

4. Discussion

Previously reported by Vale [19] indicates that he obtained the yield of the ethanol extract of the bark *Himatanthus articulatus* equivalent to 16.82% by lyophilization, in comparison with other studies [20], and obtained a yield of 3.64% from the *H. articulatus* extract [21] and 20.12% of the methanol extract of *H. drasticus* leaves by maceration.

The stress signal manifestation and "*leakage*" (increased swimming activity) were present in all concentrations even at the beginning of the experiment. Within the behavioral changes observed were increased swimming activity, tremors on the axis of the tail, loss of mobility, loss of posture, animal deposition tank bottom, and ultimately death. In addition to these manifestations, fish shallow breathing was also observed; this indicates a malfunction on the condition of the animal [22]. Other authors also report it as a defense mechanism against stressful conditions or elements present on their environment [23], which is an attempt to decrease the likelihood of death, or else there may be a metabolic cost-saving behavior to maintain the overall physiological homeostasis.

The behavioral changes described by Ribeiro [12], at the concentration of 170 μg/mL ethanolic extract of Jambu, are similar with the two highest concentrations of TPJM (1000 and 1500 μg/mL).

According to Barreto [24], the gills are especially sensitive to toxic substances dissolved in the aqueous environment because of their direct contact with the water in the gas exchange. Since Hoffman et al. [25] report that the gills are sites of potential absorption for toxic agents present in the water, and they are considered as the main site for the absorption of toxic agents, due to their characteristics such as large surface contact, the small diffusion distance, and the large countercurrent flow between water and blood.

According to Rigolim-Sá [26], the proliferation of the respiratory epithelium-like massive hyperplasia and lamellar fusion, among other changes, is the first gills' defense mechanism that promotes increased water-blood barrier enhancing the detoxification process. Epithelial proliferation is an initial response of the respiratory system. These defense mechanisms are typical because they reduce or even entirely prevent the passage of water between the secondary lamellae. This loss of respiratory surface can cause death by anoxia [27–29].

Meletti and Rocha [16] reported that the mucous cells and chloride cells might become hyperplastic and/or hypertrophic as a result of toxic agents present in the water. The presence of chloride cells and mucous cells in the secondary lamellae, as well the hypertrophy and hyperplasia, was observed at all concentrations, which demonstrate the potential change of the standard metabolism of these cell types when TPJM was administered due to proliferation expression proteins or the enhancement on their transport activity [1].

Takashima and Hibya [17] reported that many pathogenic agents might lead to epithelial swelling, vacuolization, and necrosis of secondary lamellae as observed in this study. However, this amendment undermines the primary function of the gills, whose function is to carry out the gas exchange, endangering the homeostasis of the body [16].

The hepatic metabolism of the *D. rerio* is similar to mammals and rodents. This fish metabolizes drugs using similar pathways used by humans. They have a wide range of cytochrome P-450 enzymes, allowing metabolic reactions, including hydroxylation, conjugation, oxidation, demethylation, and deethylation. Also, the liver synthesizes the bile salts, stores the glycogen, and produces vitellogenin, a protein present in the skin that surrounds the egg [30, 31].

Meletti and Rocha [16] points out that the vacuolation in hepatocytes can be an indirect measure but the not very precise amount of glycogen or lipids contained in this cell type.

Silva [32] reports that a reduction of glycogen in hepatocytes may represent the beginning of a nonspecific response to stress in fish induced by different chemical compounds. All stage I changes were present in various concentrations of treatment. It may be noted in particular the disruption of hepatic cords, loss or atypia contour of hepatocytes, intense vacuolation, and decreased glycogen like the observations shown (**Figures 7–9**).

However, the reduction of bilirubin binding capacity of this acid may explain the liver dysfunction [17, 33].

Robins and Contran [34] state that necrosis in liver tissue is related to intoxication processes, indicating that the severity of the injury is proportional to the type of, duration of the inflammation, the severity of aggression, and physiological state. Poleksic and Karan [35] observed necrosis in carp hepatocytes and exposed the importance of histopathology to analyze the damage similar to the observations with the treatment with the NSAID drug paracetamol [36].

The kidneys are the main route of excretion for metabolites of various xenobiotics on the zebrafish. It represents one of the common routes of elimination due to the urine formation and the excretion on an aqueous environment, some by glomerular filtration, others by resorption, or by secretion of processes tubular [32].

The kidneys receive large blood flow; the presence of chemicals in the blood can lead to some pathological changes in the Bowman's capsule, such as the abnormal proliferation of epithelial cells and thickening of the basal membrane, resulting in the reduction of Bowman's space. This change can impair the filtration process of the whole blood and renal function [17, 18].

The tubular obstruction is a histopathologic change of stage I. According to Meletti and Rocha [16], this change is classified as a type and "cloudy swelling," which is characterized by the presence of tubular epithelial cells or swollen with hypertrophied fine granules of eosinophils in the cytoplasm.

The hyaline degeneration was also observed at the concentrations tested. This modification is characterized by the presence of massive eosinophil granules, which according to Takashima and Hibyia [17] and Hilton and Lauren [18] can be produced inside the cell or formed by reabsorption of excess protein substances possibly formed by the glomerulus. Meletti and Rocha [16] affirms that many of the tubular changes observed in the kidneys of *D. rerio* are caused by metabolic disorders by toxic agents. Also, according to Takashima and Hibyia [17], most tubular degenerative changes are often culminating in necrosis.

The dilation of the glomerular capillaries and the glomerular degeneration were frequent changes in all groups exposed to TPJM. According to Takashima and Hibyia [17], the occurrences of these changes are manifested on pathological conditions due to changes of the basal lamina and are typically accompanied by changes in podocyte and endothelial cells, such as hyperplasia.

The occurrence of new nephrons or tubules regeneration was unusual in groups treated with TPJM (**Figure 10**). Preexisting renal tubules can often be regenerated after being damaged by some diseases or even toxic agents [17]. According to Hinton and Laurén [18], tubular regeneration in fishes can be a good indication of adaptation and recovery. Also, after kidney damage induced by toxic agents, there may be entirely new nephron production [17, 37]. However, one can find new nephrons in unpolluted water fish, without the presence of toxic or xenobiotic agents (**Figures 11** and **12**).

All this evidence provides for the first time some information of the histopathological changes on the main detoxification organs of *D. rerio* by the exposition of TPJM, although further analysis is needed to be done in order to correlate the phytochemical composition with the toxic effects or the therapeutical ones.

5. Conclusions

The exposure of *Danio rerio* in concentrations of 500, 750, 1000, and 1500 μg/mL of TPJM for 48 h concludes that the TPJM can be considered low toxicity when compared to products already tested in the same model, because their mortality and histopathological changes were observed at high concentrations, and based on the percentage of extractives TPJM which was 1.85%, LC_{50} equal to dose 475 mg/kg, and according with the traditional statement, which is 6 tablespoons/day, it can be inferred that only 0.5 g of active ingredients are ingested by an adult user per day, corresponding to a dose of 7.14 mg/kg, which is a far lethal dose, and the doses producing histopathologic lesions, demonstrating the low toxicity of TPJM. However, discretion is advised for the use of this phytopreparation due to the poisoning risks existing in high doses, especially face of health problems that are indicated (lung cancer, lymphatic cancer, intestinal worms, fever, and gastric ulcers).

Acknowledgements

The authors would like to thank CAPES (n° 3292/2013 AUXPE) and CNPq Proc. 402332/2013-0 for the financial support.

Conflict of interest

The authors declare that there are no conflicts of interest.

Author details

Igor Victor Ferreira dos Santos[1,2], Gisele Custódio de Souza[1,2], Giovanna Rocha Santana[2], Jonatas Lobato Duarte[2], Caio Pinho Fernandes[1,3], Hady Keita[2], Josué Arturo Velázquez-Moyado[4], Andrés Navarrete[4], Irlon Maciel Ferreira[1,2], Helison Oliveira Carvalho[2] and José Carlos Tavares Carvalho[1,2]*

*Address all correspondence to: farmacos@unifap.br

1 Programa de Pós-graduação em Ciências Farmacêuticas, Departamento de Ciências Biológicas e da Saúde, Universidade Federal do Amapá, Brazil

2 Laboratório de Pesquisa em Fármacos, Curso de Farmácia, Departamento de Ciências Biológicas e da Saúde, Universidade Federal do Amapá, Brazil

3 Laboratório de Nanobiotecnologia Fitofarmacêutica, Curso de Farmácia, Departamento de Ciências Biológicas e da Saúde, Universidade Federal do Amapá, Brazil

4 Facultad de Química, Departamento de Farmacia, Universidad Nacional Autónoma de México, Ciudad de México, Mexico

References

[1] Sinha AK et al. Gill remodeling in three freshwater teleosts in response to high environmental ammonia. Aquatic Toxicology. 2014;**155**:166-180

[2] Kuklinski C. Farmacognosia estudio de las drogas y sustancias medicamentosas de origen natural. Primera edición. Madrid-España: Editorial Omega S.A. de edición 2000. 2003

[3] Lorenzi H. Plantas daninhas do Brasil: Terrestres, aquáticas, parasitas e tóxicas. Instituto Plantarum de Estudos da Flora. São Paulo, SP: Nova Odessa; 2008

[4] de Mesquita ML, Desrivot J, Fournet A, de Paula JE, Grellier P, Espindola LS. Antileishmanial and trypanocidal activity of Brazilian Cerrado plants. Memórias do Instituto Oswaldo Cruz. 2005;**100**:783-787

[5] Perdue GP, Blomster RN. South American plants III: Isolation of fulvoplumierin from *Himatanthus sucuuba* (M. Arg.) Woodson (Apocynaceae). Journal of Pharmaceutical Sciences. 1978;**67**:1322-1323

[6] Colares A, Cordeiro L, Costa JGM, Silveira E, Campos A, Cardoso A. Phytochemical and biological preliminary study of Himatanthus drasticus (Mart.) Plumel (Janaguba). Pharmacognosy Magazine. 2008;**4**:73

[7] Luz HS, Santos ACG, Machado KRG. Prospecção fitoquímica de *Himatanthus drasticus* Plumel (Apocynaceae), da mesorregião leste maranhense. Revista Brasileira de Plantas Medicinais. 2014;**16**:657-662

[8] Sousa ELD, Grangeiro ARS, Bastos IVGA, Rodrigues GCR, Silva MJE, Anjos FBRD, Sousa CELD, et al. Antitumor activity of leaves of Himatanthus drasticus (Mart.) Plumel-Apocynaceae (Janaguba) in the treatment of Sarcoma 180 tumor. Brazilian Journal of Pharmaceutical Sciences. 2010;**46**(2):199-203

[9] Mousinho KC, Oliveira C de C, Ferreira JR de O, Carvalho AA, Magalhães HIF, Bezerra DP, Alves APNN, Costa-Lotufo LV, Pessoa C, de Matos MPV. Antitumor effect of laticifer proteins of *Himatanthus drasticus* (Mart.) Plumel–Apocynaceae. Journal of Ethnopharmacology. 2011;**137**:421-426

[10] Lucetti DL, Lucetti EC, Bandeira MA, Veras HN, Silva AH, Leal LK, Lopes AA, Alves VCC, Silva GS, Brito GA. Anti-inflammatory effects and possible mechanism of action of lupeol acetate isolated from Himatanthus drasticus (Mart.) Plumel. Journal of Inflammation Research. 2010;**7**:b12

[11] Zhang J, Wang ZM, Liu KC, He QX, Qi YD, Zhang BG, Liu HT, Xiao PG. Chemical constituents of Kadsura oblongifolia and evaluation of their toxicity. Yao xue xue bao = Acta Pharmaceutica Sinica. 2014;**49**:1296-1303

[12] Ribeiro LC. Investigação do efeito ictiotóxico do extrato etanólico da raíz de *Spilanthes acmella* (jambú) em zebrafish através da análise eletrofisiológica e comportamental; 2013

[13] Souza GC. Estudo da toxicidade da nanoemulsão de álcool perílico (NPOH) sobre zebrafish (Danio rerio Hamilton, 1822). Macapá: Dissertação (Mestrado); 2015

[14] Schwaiger J, Wanke R, Adam S, Pawert M, Honnen W, Triebskorn R. The use of histopathological indicators to evaluate contaminant-related stress in fish. Journal of Aquatic Ecosystem Stress and Recovery. 1997;**6**:75-86

[15] Poleksic V, Mitrovic TV. Fish Gills as Monitor of Sublethal Chronic Effects of Pollution. In: Muller R, Lloyd R, editors. Sublethal and Chronic Effects of Pollutants on Freshwater Fish. Farnham: Fishing News Books Ltd.; 1994. pp. 339-352

[16] Meletti PC, Rocha O. Avaliação da degradação ambiental na bacia do Rio Mogi-Guaçu por meio de testes de toxicidade com sedimento e de análises histopatológicas em peixes. São Carlos: UFSCAR; 2003. pp. 149-180

[17] Takashima F, Hibiya T. An Atlas of Fish Histology: Normal and Pathological Features. In: Fischer G, editor. Tokyo, Japan: Kodanska; 1995

[18] Hinton DE, Lauren DJ. Integrative histopathological approaches to detecting effects of environmental stressors on fishes. In: American Fisheries Society Symposium. 1990. Vol. 8. pp. 51-66

[19] Vale VV. Estudo fitoquímico e atividade antiplasmódica em *Plasmodium falciparum* (W2) de *Himatanthus articulatus* (Vahl) Woodson (Apocynaceae); 2014

[20] Vilhena TC. Avaliação da toxicidade dos efeitos do extrato etanólico seco das cascas de Himatanthus articulatus (Vahl) Woodson (Apocynaceae) sobre as alterações oxidativas

na malária experimental in vivo (Dissertação de mestrado PPGCF). Brazil: Universidade Federal do Pará; 2012. 139f

[21] Sousa EL. Avaliação da atividade antitumoral de *Himatanthus drasticus* (Mart.) Plumel Apocynaceae (Janaguba). Dissertação de Mestrado. CCS-UFPE. Federal University of Pernambuco. 2009

[22] Little EE, Fairchild JF, DeLonay AJ. Behavioral methods for assessing impacts of contaminants on early life stage fishes. In: American Fisheries Society Symposium. American Fisheries Society Symposium; 1993:67-76

[23] Schreck CB, Olla BL, Davis MW, Iwama GK, Pickering AD, Sumpter JP, Schreck CB. Behavioral responses to stress. Fish Stress and Health in Aquaculture. 1997;**62**:145-170

[24] Barreto T de R. Alterações morfofuncionais e metabólicas no teleósteo de água doce matrinxã, Brycon cephalus (GÜNTHER, 1869) exposto ao organofosforado metil paration (Folisuper 600 BR®) (Dissertação (Mestrado em Ciências Fisiológicas). São Paulo: Universidade Federal de São Carlos; 2007. 105 f

[25] Hoffman DJ, Rattner BA, Burton GA Jr, Cairns J Jr. Handbook of Ecotoxicology. Boca Raton, FL: CRC Press; 2002

[26] Rigolin-Sá O. Toxicidade do herbicida Roundup (glifosato) e do acaricida Omite (propargito) nas fases iniciais da ontogenia do bagre, Rhandia hilarii (Valenciennes, 1840) (Pimelodidade, Siluriformes). Tese (Doutorado em Recusos Naturais) Curso de Pós-graduação em Ecologia e Recursos Naturais. São Carlos: Universidade Federal de São Carlos; 1998. 307f

[27] Smart G. The effect of ammonia exposure on gill structure of the rainbow trout (*Salmo gairdneri*). Journal of Fish Biology. 1976;**8**:471-475

[28] Rand GM, Petrocelli SR. Fundamentals of Aquatic Toxicology: Methods and Applications. Princeton, NJ: FMC Corp.; 1985

[29] Nogueira DJ, de Castro SC, Vieira RCA, de Sá OR, de Azevedo Santos VM. Utilização das brânquias de Pimelodus maculatus (Lacèpéde, 1803) (Siluriformes; Pimelodidae) como biomarcador de poluição no reservatório da UHE Marechal Mascarenhas de Moraes, Minas Gerais, Brasil. Biotemas. 2011;**24**:51-58

[30] Vliegenthart AD, Tucker CS, Del Pozo J, Dear JW. Zebrafish as model organisms for studying drug-induced liver injury. British Journal of Clinical Pharmacology. 2014;**78**(6):1217-1227

[31] Goksoyr A, Husoy AM. Immunochemical approaches to studies of CYP1A localization and induction by xenobiotics in fish. In: Fish Ecotoxicology. Birkhäuser, Basel: Springer; 1998. p. 165-202

[32] Silva AG. Alterações histopatológicas de peixes como biomarcadores de contaminação aquática. Tese de Doutorado (Dissertação (Mestrado em Ciências Biológicas). Paraná: Universidade Estadual de Londrina; 2004. 74 p

[33] Pacheco M, Santos MA. Biotransformation, genotoxic, and histopathological effects of environmental contaminants in European eel (*Anguilla anguilla* L.). Ecotoxicology and Environmental Safety. 2002;**53**:331-347

[34] Robins C, Cotran RS. Patologia—Bases patológicas das doenças. 7ª. edição: Elsevier; 2005

[35] Poleksic V, Karan V. Effects of trifluralin on carp: Biochemical and histological evaluation. Ecotoxicology and Environmental Safety. 1999;**43**:213-221

[36] North TE, Goessling W, Walkley CR, Lengerke C, Kopani KR, Lord AM, Weber GJ, Bowman TV, Jang IH, Grosser T, Fitzgerald GA, Daley GQ, Orkin SH, Zon LI. Prostaglandin E2 regulates vertebrate hematopoietic stem cell homeostasis. Nature. 2007;**447**:1007-1011

[37] Reimschuessel R. A fish model of renal regeneration and development. ILAR Journal. 2001;**42**:285-291

Section 2

Head and Neck Tumors

Chapter 4

Histopathology of the Ocular Surface

Hind Alkatan and Tariq Alzahem

Additional information is available at the end of the chapter

http://dx.doi.org/10.5772/intechopen.75066

Abstract

Three integral parts that cover the ocular surface are the conjunctiva, limbus, and cornea. The conjunctiva is a see-through mucous membrane that lines the internal surface of the eyelids and the front surface of the eyeball, ending at the limbus. It is highly vascular with a dense lymphatic network. The limbus forms the boundary between the transparent cornea and the opaque sclera. The cornea is a complex structure that provides a protective function and is responsible for about 75% of the optical power of the eye. Histology of these highly specialized biological materials as well as the ways in which individual components are structurally and functionally related will be discussed in this chapter. Then, we will go over the pathological oncology processes that can affect the ocular surface.

Keywords: histology, histopathology, ocular surface, conjunctiva, limbus, cornea, epithelium, stroma, endothelium, squamous cell carcinoma, melanoma

1. Introduction

The ocular surface is an anatomic entity that is composed of different ocular structures: conjunctiva, limbus, and cornea. A healthy ocular surface should have a healthy tear film overlying it. The maintenance of ocular surface in an optimal and healthy state contributes both esthetic and functional wellness of the eye.

From the anatomic point of view, the ocular surface includes the mucosal epithelium limited by the skin of the free edge of the eyelids. It includes the cornea and the conjunctiva. The interdependence of the structures integrated into this system and their influence on the corneal epithelium and ultimately on the eyeball makes them of great importance to the health of the eye. In addition, the primordial cells of the corneal epithelium are located at the corneoscleral limbus.

Tumors of the conjunctiva can arise from any of the cells that are naturally present and are evident histologically; thus, there is a wide variety of these tumors. They originate from the squamous epithelium, melanocytes, and lymphocytic cells found in the conjunctival stroma. The epithelial and melanocytic origins are more frequent.

This chapter will start by describing the normal histology of the ocular surface with selected correlated functional aspects of the biologic micro-design. Afterward, the most important malignant neoplastic processes affecting the conjunctiva will be reviewed along with the latest updates in the medical literature.

2. Histology of ocular surface

2.1. Conjunctiva

The conjunctiva is a transparent mucous membrane that covers the ocular surface from the limbus to the mucocutaneous junction. It plays an essential role in maintaining a healthy and optically clear cornea. The part covering the sclera is known as the bulbar conjunctiva, while the palpebral conjunctiva lines the posterior surface of the eyelids. The forniceal conjunctiva is the portion that connects the bulbar with the palpebral parts. The bulbar conjunctiva is loosely attached to the underlying Tenon's capsule except at the limbus where they fuse together. The palpebral part is tightly adherent to the tarsus, while the forniceal portion is loose and redundant. A crescent-shaped fold of the conjunctiva called the plica semilunaris is found nasally. Medial to the plica lies the caruncle, a pinkish globular nodule that contains sebaceous glands and hair follicles in addition to the adnexal elements of the conjunctival stroma.

The surface layer of the conjunctiva is composed of non-keratinizing stratified squamous epithelium with numerous goblet cells. Melanocytes are normally present in the basal layer of the epithelium. The morphology and the number of layers of the conjunctival epithelial cells change according to the region from which a biopsy was taken. There are approximately six to nine layers of stratified squamous epithelium in the bulbar conjunctiva. The epithelial cells are columnar in the forniceal part and cuboidal in the area attached to the tarsus where the epithelial cells are packed in two to five layers. The goblet cells are distributed throughout the bulbar and tarsal conjunctiva and are most concentrated inferonasally and in the region of the caruncle and plica semilunaris.

The conjunctival stroma (substantia propria) is a thin, richly vascularized layer enclosing scattered lacrimal glands (based on the anatomic location), lymphatics, plasma cells, macrophages, and mast cells. Additionally, it comprises numerous elastic fibers that facilitate globe movement in all gazes. Specialized collections of T and B lymphocytes underlying a modified epithelium is known as conjunctiva-associated lymphoid tissue (CALT). It functions to process antigens and provides immunity against pathologic microbes on the ocular surface [1]. Conjunctival stem cells are scattered throughout the bulbar or forniceal conjunctiva.

2.2. Corneoscleral limbus

The limbus is the transitional region between the corneal margin and the anterior sclera. It is approximately 1–1.5 mm wide. The limbus contains the corneal stem cells located in the basal cell layer. There are histological, pathological, and surgical definitions of the limbus. Histologically, the central margin of the limbus is limited by a line connecting the peripheral termination of Bowman's layer externally and Schwalbe's line, the peripheral termination of Descemet's membrane, internally. The peripheral margin of the limbus is bounded by the central margin of the scleral spur. The peripheral margin from pathologist's point of view is formed by a vertical line that is perpendicular to the scleral spur [1].

Surgically, the limbus is divided into two zones: a central blue-gray zone and a peripheral white zone. The central zone corresponds to the area connecting Bowman's layer and Descemet's membrane. The peripheral zone overlies the trabecular meshwork [2].

2.3. Cornea

The cornea is the anterior and transparent portion of the fibrous tunic of the eye globe and is the most powerful refractive element of the optical system of the eye. Its transparency is a function of different factors: avascularity, relative acellularity, relative dehydration, and the remarkable organization of the stromal collagen lamellae. The anterior surface of the cornea measures 11–12 mm horizontally and 10–11 mm vertically. The thickness of the cornea is 0.52 mm centrally and 0.65 mm peripherally. The water content is 78% and is controlled by intact epithelium and endothelium. Its refractive index is 1.376 [1].

In the following sections, the histology of the different layers of the cornea will be described from anterior to posterior: the epithelium, Bowman's layer, stroma, Descemet's membrane, and endothelium.

2.3.1. Epithelium

The corneal epithelium is the outermost layer of the cornea and is derived from the embryonic surface ectoderm. It is composed of 4–5 multilayered stratified, non-keratinized squamous epithelium with an underlying single layer of basal cells. It is continuous with the conjunctival epithelium at the limbus. Its overall thickness is approximately 50 μm with a complete turnover in 7–10 days. This multilayered epithelium is distributed in three strata: superficial flattened cells, middle wing cells, and deep basal cells [1].

The basal cell layer is considered the mother of the overlying cells, i.e., wing and the superficial cells. The basal cell density is approximately 6000 cells/mm^2. They originate from the corneal limbal stem cells. The new cells travel from the limbus in a centripetal manner at a rate of approximately 120 μm/week. The cells communicate with each other through gab junctions and actively secrete their basal lamina (50 nm thick, type IV collagen) where they adhere to it via hemidesmosomes. Alteration of hemidesmosomes can result in recurrent epithelial erosions, as seen in patients with epithelial basement membrane dystrophy (EBMD) [1].

Wing cell layer is composed of 2–3 cell rows that overly the basal cells. These cells are given this name because they have extensions that make them resemble wings in cross section. They are attached to each other by zonulae occludentes that form a semipermeable membrane, an important factor preventing components of the tear film to get into the corneal stroma. The outermost layer is 2–3 rows of flattened cells that are shed in the tear film to be replaced by other cells. The ultrastructure of their apical surfaces is rough and quite irregular owing to the presence of countless microplicae and microvilli. All epithelial cells are connected to each other by desmosomes and communicate via gap junctions. Reduction of the number of desmosomes is noted in patients with topical anesthetic abuse [3].

Growth factors secreted by the lacrimal glans and corneal epithelial cells play an essential role in the maintenance of healthy epithelial cells. Among which, insulin-like growth factor (IGF-1) and its receptor IGF-1R alterations have been implicated in cases of hyperglycemia with resultant diabetic keratopathy. This disease is associated with superficial punctate keratitis, recurrent corneal erosions, and persistent epithelial defects in addition to severe neuroepithelial dysfunction. Moreover, the interaction of IGF-1R with its twin insulin receptor (INSR) to form a hybrid receptor (the Hybrid-R) has been reported. The Hybrid-R was detected in the corneal epithelial cell nuclei where it interacts with DNA and is proposed to control gene expression important in maintaining ocular surface biology [4].

2.3.2. Bowman's layer

Bowman's layer lies directly underneath the basal lamina. As the name implies, this stratum is a layer and not a true membrane with the absence of staining by periodic acid-Schiff (PAS) stain. It is an acellular layer that cannot regenerate forming a scar after injury. It has a thickness of 8–12 μm. Similar to the corneal stroma, it is composed of type I and type V collagen, but in contrast to the stroma, the ratio of type V to type I is higher. In addition, unlike the stroma, the collagen lamellae are smaller and more randomly arranged. The limbus starts at the peripheral termination of this layer [1].

Bowman's layer is a key factor in maintaining the corneal biomechanical properties by its stiff and tough nature. Abnormalities of this layer can result in corneal ecstatic disorders such as keratoconus due to biomechanical failure [5].

2.3.3. Stroma

The corneal stroma occupies 90–95% of the thickness of the cornea. It is derived from the neural crest cells. In the center, it measures about 500 μm, while it becomes thicker toward the periphery. It is formed by proteoglycans (keratan sulfate and dermatan sulfate) covalently linked to a nucleus of a protein and a large number of collagen fibrils arranged parallel to the surface of the cornea. These corneal stromal collagen lamellae (200–250 lamellae) are composed principally of type I and type V, with lesser amounts of types III and VI. The distance between these lamellae, occupied by proteoglycans, is constant. This property is very important in maintaining the corneal transparency by eliminating any interference with light transmission [1]. A relatively recently introduced layer, the pre-Descemet's layer (Dua's layer), is an acellular layer measuring approximately 10 μm and is found in the posterior stroma [6]. Among these collagen fibrils, we find the keratocytes, which are specialized fibroblasts that synthesize collagen and proteoglycans. There are about 2.4 million keratocytes spread within the stroma with higher density being anterior. They are extremely active cells evident by abundant mitochondria, rough endoplasmic reticulum, and Golgi apparatuses. They are flat and evenly distributed. Their plasma membranes are fenestrated. Gap junctions are the conduits through which communication occurs. The cell density decreases with age at a slower rate than the corneal endothelium [1].

The posterior portion of the stroma is typically wetter than the anterior one. This occurs because of the wetting effect of the aqueous humor posteriorly and the drying effect of the atmosphere anteriorly. Corneal stromal edema, as seen in cases of endothelial failure, will result in enlarged spacing between the lamellae and subsequent visual compromise [1].

2.3.4. *Descemet's membrane*

Descemet's membrane corresponds to the basal lamina of the corneal endothelium. It is a true basement membrane that is PAS-positive. Its thickness is variable and linked to the age of the individual as it is continuously secreted by the endothelium. In neonates, it measures 2–4 μm thick and reaches up to 10–12 μm by adulthood [1]. It has two histologically distinct layers: the anterior banded layer produced in utero and the posterior non-banded layer produced throughout life. It is composed of type IV collagen, laminin, and fibronectin [1].

Descemet's membrane is fundamental in providing support and adhesion to the endothelial cells. In addition, it is resistant to the phagocytic, toxic, and enzymatic insults. However, it is relatively weakly attached to the overlying stroma and, thus, can be surgically dissected as one piece [1].

2.3.5. *Endothelium*

The corneal endothelium is a monolayer located on the inner side of the cornea and is about 4–6 μm thick. Similar to the stroma, the endothelium comes from neural crest cells. The cells cannot regenerate after birth. The endothelial cell density is about 3000 cells/mm^2 with 500,000 cells covering the posterior surface of the cornea. This number decreases slowly with age at a rate of 0.6% per year. The most common cell shape is hexagonal. Minimal variation in cell size (polymegathism) and cell shape (pleomorphism) can be seen in normal individuals. The endothelium has two principal functions aiming to maintain the corneal clarity: the barrier and the metabolic pump functions [1]. These cells are joined together by interdigitations that are only visible by an electron microscope. In addition, focal tight junctions can be seen in the apicolateral membranes. They communicate through gap junctions. The endothelial cell layer is relatively semipermeable to allow some nutrients to pass paracellularly to the remaining corneal layers [1].

The high metabolic demand of the endothelial cells is evident by the presence of numerous mitochondria, the prominent smooth and rough endoplasmic reticulum, ribosomes, and Golgi apparatuses. Pinocytic vesicles can be seen in the cytoplasm pumping fluid from the stroma to the anterior chamber [1]. The endothelial pump requires the existence of bicarbonate, the membrane bicarbonate transporters, Na-K ATPase, and carbonic anhydrase activity. Thus, corneas with low or relatively dysfunctional endothelial cells contraindicate the use of topical carbonic anhydrase inhibitors [4].

Peripheral corneal guttae (Hassall-Henle bodies) are minute excrescences that can be observed in the peripheral part of Descemet's membrane. It is considered a natural aging process. They represent focal thickening of Descemet's membrane. A histologically similar but pathological in nature is the appearance of central cornea guttae. They are associated with progressive corneal stromal and epithelial edema representing Fuch's endothelial dystrophy [1].

3. Histopathology of ocular surface

Tumors of the ocular surface are the most frequent of the eye and appendages along with those of the eyelids. They cover a wide spectrum from benign lesions such as papilloma to others that may endanger the visual function and the life of the patient, such as squamous cell carcinoma and melanoma [6, 7]. They can arise from any of the cells that make up the conjunctiva although the most frequent are those of epithelial and melanocytic origins. The tumors of the conjunctiva can be epithelial (non-melanocytic and melanocytic) and stromal (lymphoproliferative, vascular, neural, lipomatous, histiocytic, myogenic, fibrous, and choristomatous). In addition, tumors of the ocular surface encompass caruncular and metastatic tumors. This chapter will focus on the epithelial tumors.

3.1. Non-melanocytic epithelial tumors

3.1.1. Squamous papilloma

Squamous papilloma appears at any age with variable presentation [8]. Human papilloma viruses (HPV) 6, 11, or 16 result in the development of squamous papillomas in children [9]. Patients can present with pink, single or multiple, sessile, or pedunculated lesion in the inferior fornix and less commonly the bulbar conjunctiva. In older patients, papilloma can result in relation to HPV infection or in patients with compromised immunity [10]. Clinically, it usually presents as unilateral light pink mass at the limbus or the caruncle. It may have the appearance of squamous cell carcinoma (SCC). In addition, squamous papilloma is a premalignant lesion and has been reported to transform to SCC, transitional cell carcinoma, or mucoepidermoid carcinoma particularly in the inverted growth pattern [11–13]. The lesion classically demonstrates many vascularized papillary fronds lined by the acanthotic epithelium with no evidence of pleomorphism or dysplasia (**Figure 1**).

3.1.2. Conjunctival pseudoepitheliomatous hyperplasia

This lesion is a benign inflammatory lesion manifested by a reactive proliferation of the conjunctival epithelium. It is also called pseudocarcinomatous hyperplasia as it resembles malignant lesions in clinical and histopathological examinations [7]. It is caused by irritation of the conjunctiva by a coexisting or previously existing stromal inflammation, foreign body, vernal keratoconjunctivitis, pterygium, and pinguecula. Clinically, a rapidly progressing elevated pink limbal lesion with leukoplakia and hyperkeratosis is seen. The histopathology shows an extensive acanthosis and hyperkeratosis in addition to parakeratosis of the conjunctival epithelium. There is no cytological atypia.

3.1.3. Keratoacanthoma

It is a rare variant of conjunctival pseudoepitheliomatous hyperplasia. A rapidly progressing hyperkeratotic lesion is seen [8, 14–16]. The documented cases have occurred on the bulbar conjunctiva, within the palpebral aperture, and adjacent to the limbus.

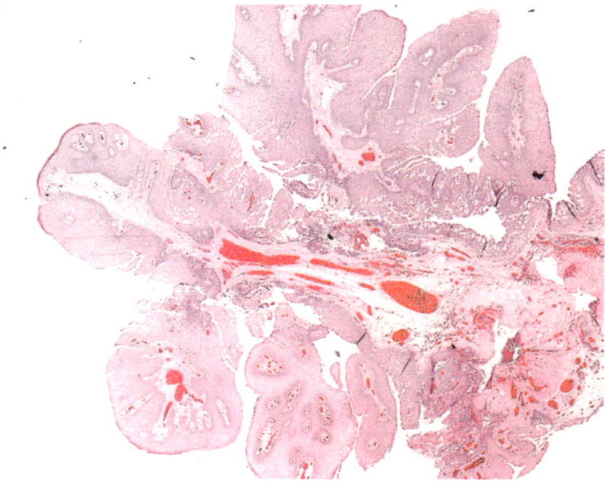

Figure 1. Histopathological image of a conjunctival squamous papilloma (original magnification ×50 hematoxylin and eosin).

3.1.4. Dacryoadenoma

Dacryoadenoma is an exceedingly rare condition occurring in children and adolescents. It is a benign tumor originating from the conjunctival epithelium and grows into the stroma forming glandular lobules analogous to the lacrimal gland with goblet cells. Clinically, it appears as a translucent fleshy lesion anywhere in the conjunctiva [8, 12, 17].

3.1.5. Conjunctival keratotic plaque and actinic keratosis

These leukoplakic conjunctival lesions cannot be differentiated clinically. They usually arise in the interpalpebral region. Histologically, a conjunctival keratotic plaque is characterized by acanthosis, hyperkeratosis, and parakeratosis. There is no dyskeratosis. Typically, it has no malignant potential.

In actinic keratosis, a gradually progressing flat leukoplakic lesion that may frequently be indistinguishable from conjunctival intra-epithelial neoplasia (CIN) is observed [8, 12, 18]. Positive rose bengal staining of the lesion surface is seen in cases of CIN. Epithelial hyperplasia acanthosis, keratosis, or parakeratosis are found in addition to some atypia. The basement membrane is intact.

3.1.6. Ocular surface squamous neoplasia (OSSN)

Ocular surface squamous neoplasia (OSSN) is a common term that describes a spectrum of benign, premalignant, and malignant epithelial lesions of the conjunctiva and cornea. Thus, OSSN encompasses conjunctival or corneal intraepithelial dysplasia, carcinoma in situ, and invasive squamous cell carcinoma (SCC) [19]. Previously, the terms used to describe the spectrum of OSSN were Bowen's disease, Bowenoid epithelioma, and intraepithelial epithelioma [20].

CIN approximately accounts for 4% of all conjunctival lesions and 39% of premalignant and malignant lesions of the ocular surface [21]. The incidence of invasive SCC is ranging from

0.02 to 3.5/100,000 population [22]. Three quarters of cases occur in men and older patients and at the limbus, although any part of the conjunctiva or cornea may be affected mostly within the interpalpebral fissure [12, 21].

Risk factors associated with the development of OSSN are exposure to sunlight, HPV type 16 infections, and immunodeficiency [12, 23]. In addition, xeroderma pigmentosum and Papillon-Lefevre syndrome are associated with recurrent OSSN, occurring in younger individuals [24]. Rarely, OSSN can be bilateral in immunosuppressed patients. Regional lymph node involvement and infrequently distant metastasis may occur.

Clinically, the lesion may appear fleshy, gelatinous, leukoplakic, or papillomatous. Leukoplakia is most likely due to hyperkeratosis or surface keratinization. Feeder vessels may be prominent, or the lesion may be avascular. As mentioned earlier, rose bengal staining can support the diagnosis and help in the demarcation of the tumor extent. It is essential to examine the tarsal conjunctiva with upper eyelid eversion to look for extension or multifocal involvement. Clinical correlation with histological severity is unpredictable. Intraocular extension occurs in 2–15% of SCC patients for which enucleation and sometimes exenteration, if the orbit is invaded by the malignant process resulting in proptosis, are often needed [22, 25]. The limbal lesion may invade the adjacent corneal epithelium and appear as advancing superficial faint opacity that may be associated with subtle vascularization. Rarely, primary SCC of the cornea can occur. Additionally, there are no reliable clinical measures for characterizing the differences between CIN and invasive SCC. However, leukoplakia raises the suspicion of malignancy and is generally absent or insignificant in CIN. Extensive vascularity and nodularity of the lesion are in favor of SCC. Tumor thickness is not a reliable sign of malignant potential, as there are thick tumors that remain confined within the epithelium. Diffuse conjunctival involvement can masquerade as conjunctivitis-type symptoms and signs [26].

The typical cytological features that are seen in OSSN on impression cytology include pleomorphic cells with hyperchromatic nuclei having an irregular outline and prominent nucleoli. However, the diagnosis of OSSN using this tool is controversial as the previously mentioned features might not be seen in the superficial layers overlying the tumor [27]. Thus, it is less sensitive in regard to the diagnosis of SCC. In addition, it cannot differentiate between CIN and invasive SCC. Hence, biopsy in suspected cases is advisable [28].

The histopathological examination of an incisional or excisional biopsy is of central role in OSSN diagnosis and treatment plan. The submitted conjunctival tissue is flattened with the mucosal surface directed upward using a filter paper with special attention to the proper orientation of the specimen. After being left to dry, it is placed in 10% buffered formalin [19]. Histopathologically, the lesion can show any of the following spectra: conjunctival epithelial dysplasia in which dysplastic cells are confined to the basal epithelial layer and/or carcinoma in situ where the full thickness of the epithelium is occupied by dysplastic cells with characteristic abrupt demarcation between the dysplastic epithelium and the normal epithelium (**Figures 2** and **3**). Invasive squamous cell carcinoma occurs when the underlying basement membrane is violated (**Figure 4**). The first two are sometimes termed conjunctival/corneal intraepithelial neoplasia (CCIN). The dysplasia is further classified into mild, moderate, and severe grades based on the level of epithelial thickness involvement. Mild dysplasia shows dysplastic cells in the lower one-third of the epithelium, while moderate dysplasia is

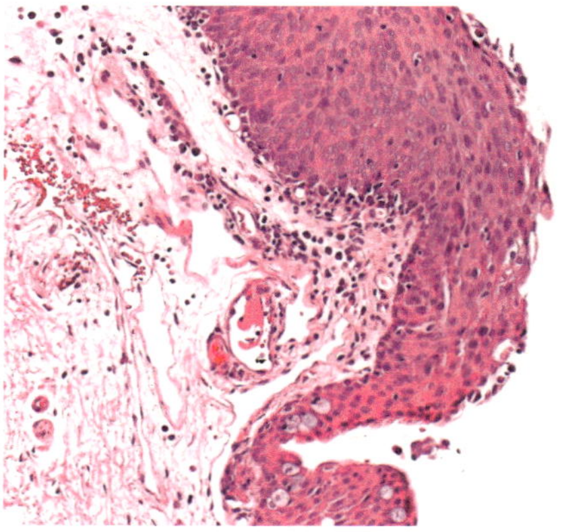

Figure 2. A case of conjunctival squamous cell carcinoma in situ with a transition from normal conjunctival epithelium to the dysplastic epithelium (original magnification ×200 hematoxylin and eosin).

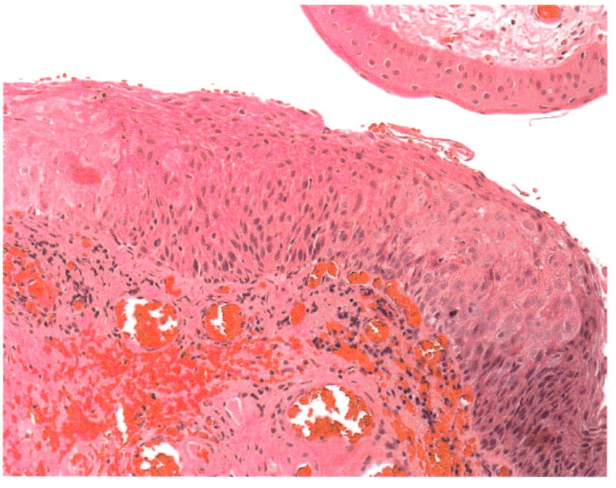

Figure 3. Another case of conjunctival squamous cell carcinoma in situ with intact basement membrane and adjacent area of normal conjunctival epithelium (original magnification ×200 hematoxylin and eosin).

involving the lower two-thirds. The histological characteristics of epithelial dysplasia include loss of polarity, increased nuclear-cytoplasmic ratio, increased number of mitotic figures, cellular polymorphism, nuclear hyperchromatism, and enlarged nucleoli. Conjunctival SCC that closely resembles the structure of the normal epithelium with keratinization is described as being well-differentiated. A tumor that resembles the original tissue to a lesser extent is termed poorly differentiated.

Increasing age, large size tumors, involvement of the surgical margins, and high Ki-67 proliferation index are risk factors for recurrence of OSSN [25]. Fortunately, with the invention of new treatment modalities, the prognosis has improved with an overall recurrence rate of approximately 5% and regional lymph node metastasis of less than 2% [19].

SCC is classified depending on the size, tumor location, and the extent of involvement as per the American Joint Committee on Cancer (AJCC) with consideration to the primary tumor

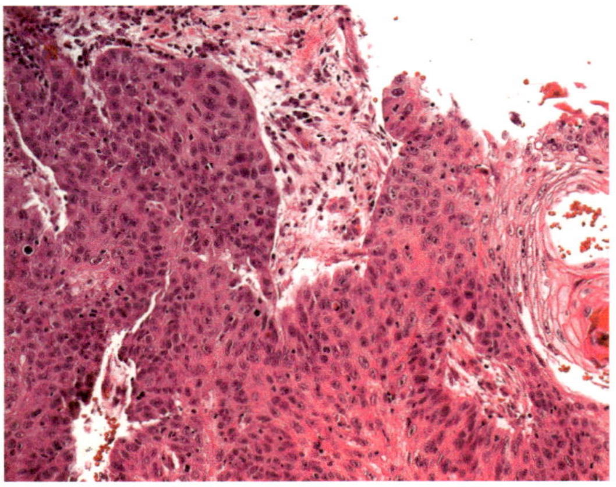

Figure 4. A case of conjunctival invasive squamous cell carcinoma with superficial keratinization (original magnification ×200 hematoxylin and eosin).

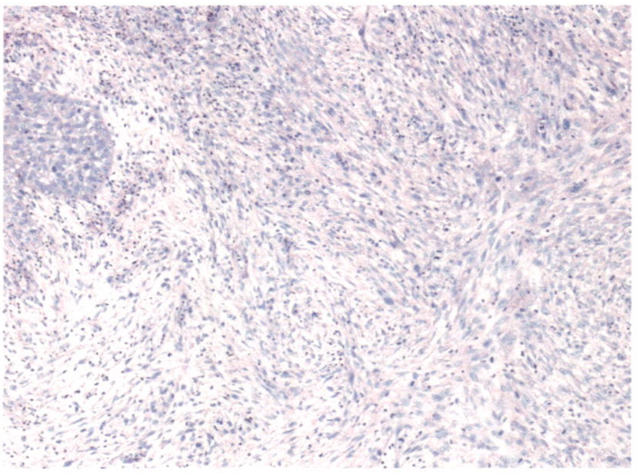

Figure 5. A case of conjunctival spindle cell carcinoma with wavy pattern of spindle cells and high degree of pleomorphism (original magnification ×100 Periodic acid-Schiff).

features, lymph node involvement, and metastasis represented using (TNM) classification. Highly malignant variants include spindle cell squamous carcinoma (**Figure 5**), mucoepidermoid carcinoma, and adenoid SCC [8, 12, 23, 29, 30, 31].

The concept of molecular genetics in cases of OSSN and ocular oncology has expanded in the recent years. It studies the interaction between genes and protein with attention to the activity patterns in different neoplastic cells. Alterations on chromosome 8 with 8p11.22 amplifications have been described in 75% of the tumors. This region encompasses a group of genes that code for ADAM proteins. One of the genes in this group is involved in oral SCC. In addition, Collagen type I alpha1 (COL1A1) is also found in ocular cases and was identified to be upregulated in oral squamous cell carcinoma [32, 33].

3.2. Melanocytic epithelial tumors

Melanocytic conjunctival lesions have a wide spectrum of disorders. They range from benign to highly malignant fatal tumors. In the following subsections, the most common differential diagnoses of melanocytic conjunctival lesions will be discussed.

3.2.1. Conjunctival nevus

Conjunctival nevi are the most common melanocytic conjunctival tumors. Conjunctival nevi usually start to appear in children or adolescents as a group of pigmented cells in the basal layer of the conjunctival epithelium. Conjunctival nevi are more prevalent in Caucasians (89%) with Africans (6%) and Asians (5%) being less commonly affected [33]. Conjunctival nevi are typically pigmented, but approximately 16% can be amelanotic or partially pigmented [12, 34]. Juxta-limbal location is the most common location occurring in more than two-thirds of patients. Other locations include the caruncle, plica semilunaris, fornix, tarsus, and cornea [34, 35].

There are three types of conjunctival nevi based on their histological location: compound, subepithelial, and junctional nevi being the least common. Compound nevi are characterized by the presence of melanocytic cells at the epithelial-subepithelial junction and within the stroma (**Figure 6**). Subepithelial lesions are located solely in the subepithelial area. They are often associated with epithelial inclusions cysts and goblet cells (**Figure 7**). Junctional nevi consist of nests of nevus cells at the epithelial-subepithelial junction. They are rare except in children. These types are considered more of phases of migration of the nevus cells from the basal epithelium to the conjunctival stroma.

Malignant transformation was estimated to be <1% [21, 35]. However, new onset in middle age or later in life, unusual location (i.e., fornix, tarsus, caruncle, plica), large lesions more than 10 mm in diameter, prominent feeder vessel or intrinsic vascularity with hemorrhage, non-cystic lesions, and non-mobile lesions (i.e., fixed to the underlying episclera) are clinical indications to excise the lesion [36].

3.2.2. Complexion-associated melanosis (CAM)

CAM, also known as racial melanosis, is a benign bilateral conjunctival lesion found among darkly pigmented individuals [8, 12]. It is typically observed in the peri-limbal area and uncommonly in the fornix or palpebral conjunctiva. On examination, variably pigmented non-cystic flat lesions are observed.

3.2.3. Primary acquired melanosis (PAM)

PAM is defined as melanocytic proliferation in the conjunctival epithelium. It is more frequent in light-skinned individuals and is usually unilateral. It typically begins insidiously in the middle age. Sunlight exposure may be a risk factor in the development of PAM. It may originate from an abnormality in neural crest as it has also been seen in patients with neurofibromatosis [37].

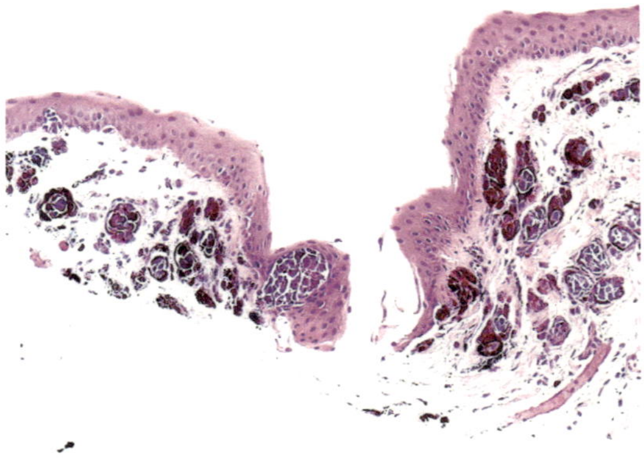

Figure 6. Histopathological appearance of a compound conjunctival nevus with nests of nevus cells at the base of the conjunctival epithelium and within the substantia propria (original magnification ×50 hematoxylin and eosin).

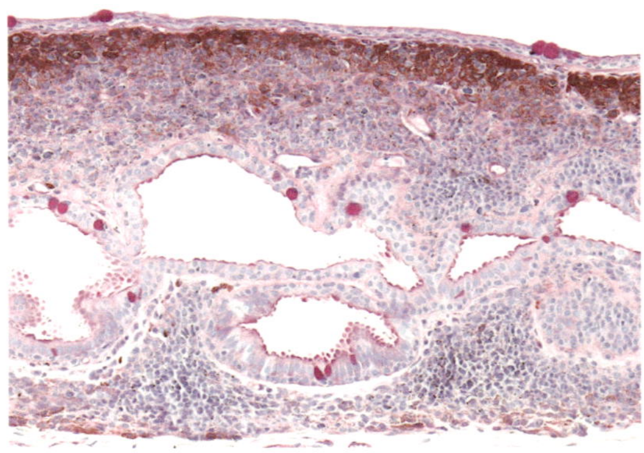

Figure 7. Histopathological appearance of a subepithelial conjunctival nevus with cystic areas lined by the conjunctival epithelium and goblet cells within the substantia propria (original magnification ×100 periodic acid-Schiff).

It presents as a flat brown, superficial, non-cystic, solitary, patchy, diffuse, or multifocal pigmentation involving bulbar, forniceal, and palpebral conjunctiva or cornea. Amelanotic PAM can be occasionally seen [8, 21, 38]. Cellular atypia, determined by biopsy and careful histopathological examination, aided by immunohistochemical staining (using Melan-A stain to highlight the melanocytes), is the principal risk factor for progression to melanoma (**Figures 8** and **9**). In one study of 311 eyes with PAM, lesions without atypia or with mild atypia demonstrated 0% progression into melanoma. On the other hand, 13% of patients having PAM with severe atypia progressed into melanoma [21].

Clinical indications to perform a biopsy include ≥5 mm lesion diameter, progression, thickening, the appearance of a nodule, vascularity, involvement of the palpebral conjunctiva or cornea, patients with personal or family history of dysplastic nevus syndrome, and history of ocular or extraocular melanoma [12].

http://dx.doi.org/10.5772/intechopen.75066

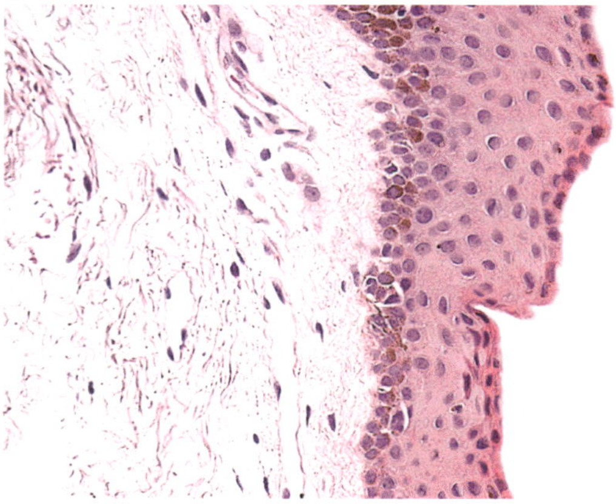

Figure 8. Histopathological appearance of conjunctival primary acquired melanosis (PAM) with melanocytic proliferation at the base of the conjunctival epithelium without evidence of atypia (original magnification ×200 hematoxylin and eosin).

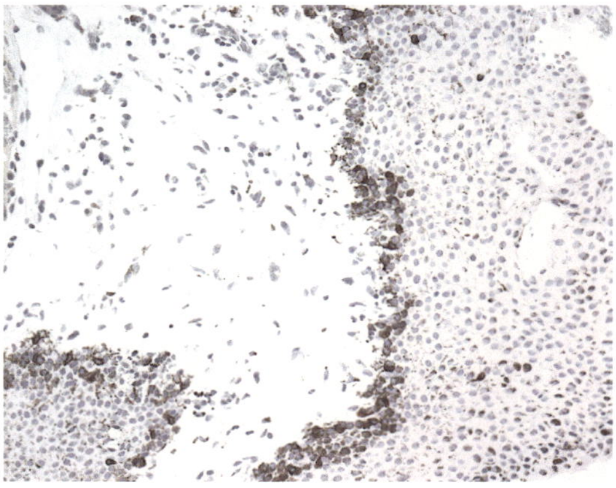

Figure 9. Immunohistochemical staining of another case of conjunctival primary acquired melanosis (PAM) showing clearly the melanocytic proliferation at the base of the conjunctival epithelium without evidence of atypia (original magnification ×200 Melan-A).

3.2.4. Conjunctival melanoma

Conjunctival melanoma, although rare, represents the second most frequent malignant conjunctival lesion after squamous cell carcinoma [39]. In the past, its evolution almost invariably resulted in an unfavorable prognosis, resulting in orbital exenteration in an attempt to eradicate the highly invasive disease. It represents a challenge for the clinician and pathologist because it can present in several pictures and originates from apparently benign lesions such as conjunctival nevi [40]. Conjunctival melanoma most frequently affects white individuals with an incidence varying from 0.24 to 0.80/1,000,000 population [41, 42]. It is more frequent in elderly individuals with a mean age ranging from 55 to 70 years [41–47]. Although rare in young people, there are reports of conjunctival melanoma cases in patients less than 20 years of age [48, 49]. There is no significant difference between men and women [41–47].

Conjunctival melanoma arises from PAM in 75% of cases, preexisting nevus in 20%, and de novo in 5% [8, 12]. Systemic risk factors include dysplastic nevus syndrome, neurofibromatosis, and xeroderma pigmentosum [38]. Sunlight exposure is also suggested as a cause in the development of bulbar conjunctival melanoma. The most frequent location of conjunctival melanoma is the bulbar conjunctiva in the peri-limbal area, but it can occur in any location, such as the palpebral or forniceal conjunctiva, the plica, or the region of the caruncle [45, 47, 50, 51].

Clinically, conjunctival melanomas may have variable presentations. Classically, it presents as a mass or an elevated pigmented conjunctival lesion. In some cases, it may appear more diffuse or multiple, with poorly defined borders, particularly when associated with PAM [22]. Less commonly, conjunctival melanomas can present as a pink or reddish pigmented lesion or can be even amelanotic, making it difficult to recognize and, thus, delaying its diagnosis and treatment [47]. Moreover, the recurrence of conjunctival melanoma after excision is typically amelanotic [12]. Repeated and continuous contact of the conjunctiva from an adjacent eyelid margin melanoma may cause a secondary conjunctival melanoma (implantation melanoma) [52]. Like SCC, conjunctival melanoma is classified according to the AJCC-TNM classification. Conjunctival melanomas can metastasize regionally to pre-auricular and submandibular lymph nodes. Distant metastasis involves the brain, liver, skin, and bone [53].

Conjunctival melanocytic intra-epithelial neoplasia (C-MIN) is a term used to describe lesions exhibiting proliferation of melanocytes. Scoring of C-MIN is based on several factors including the pattern of horizontal and vertical epithelial involvement, the degree of cellular atypia, nuclear and cellular diameter, and the presence of nucleoli and mitotic figures. Then, C-MIN is graded from 0 to 10 with 0 corresponding to an absence of any melanocytic proliferation or atypia (i.e., melanosis only), 1–4 corresponding to the severity of PAM (i.e., mild, moderate, and severe atypia), and 5–10 corresponding to conjunctival melanoma in situ (**Figure 10**) [54].

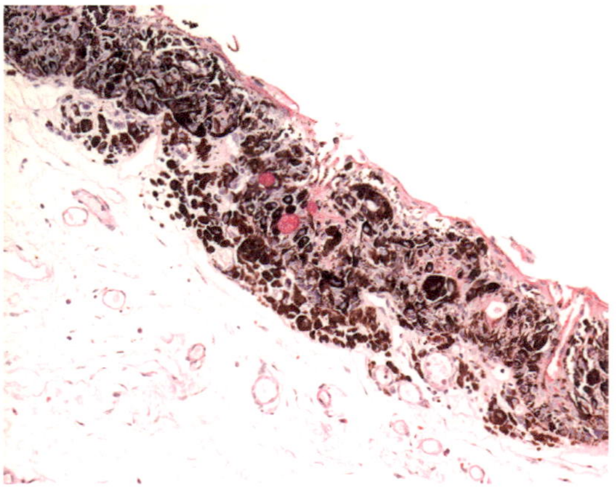

Figure 10. Histopathological appearance of conjunctival melanoma in situ with atypical melanocytic proliferation involving the full thickness of the conjunctival epithelium (original magnification ×200 periodic acid-Schiff).

The lesions usually demonstrate atypical melanocytic proliferation characterized by abundant cytoplasm, prominent nucleoli, and atypical mitotic figures with invasion of the underlying conjunctival stroma as well as the adjacent epithelium. Atypical melanocytic proliferation can be limited to the epithelium in the early stages in cases arising from PAM (melanoma in situ) with radial spread in a similar way to cutaneous melanomas. The entire lesion should be removed in one piece without touching it by excising it along the limbus to prevent seeding of the tumor cells in the surgical area.

Pathological examination of the excised lesion should include observation of important features such as ulceration, thickness of the tumor and its predominant histologic cell type (i.e., epithelioid or spindle), and the vertical growth phase. Other important characteristics include lymphocytic infiltration, vascular or perineural invasion, and the mitotic activity detected using Ki-67 index. In addition, microscopic satellitosis—defined as separate nests of tumor disconnected from the main malignant mass—should be also observed [55].

Evident histopathological features that are associated with worse survival include tumor thickness more than 2 mm, the presence of ulceration, epithelioid morphology, higher count of mitotic figures ($>1/mm^2$), lymphovascular invasion, and microsatellitosis [55, 56]. Extrabulbar conjunctival melanoma is found in a multivariate analysis study to be associated with poor outcome [57].

Immunohistochemical (IHC) stains for melanocytes such as Melan-A red, MART-1, S-100 protein, HMB-45, and the cell proliferative marker Ki-67 may help to identify melanocytic problematic cases. In conjunctival melanomas, the immunohistochemical expression of HMB-45 and Ki-67 is higher than what is observed in PAM or conjunctival nevi [58]. Beta-catenin is an IHC marker that was more strongly expressed in conjunctival melanomas compared to nevi and PAM. Thus, its role in conjunctival melanomas is different than cutaneous melanoma, in which loss of beta-catenin expression has been associated with a more aggressive course [58]. Programmed cell death protein 1 (PD-1) and its interaction with its ligand PD-L1 studied in patients with conjunctival melanoma has shown increased risk of distant metastases and worse survival when expressed by the tumor [59].

BRAF is a human gene that encodes a protein called B-Raf, a proto-oncogene. Conjunctival melanoma is one of the BRAF mutation-associated malignancies. A higher chance of distant metastasis might be seen in conjunctival melanomas expressing BRAF mutations. Conjunctival melanoma and cutaneous melanoma show resemblance in the significance of this type of mutation and its relevance to the clinical presentation [57, 60].

Advanced therapy of conjunctival melanomas using cryotherapy, radiotherapy, and chemotherapy has lowered the frequency of surgical exenteration. It is essential to perform periodic systemic screening in high-risk patients [54]. Local recurrence after therapy ranges from 50 to 70% at 10 years with an overall mortality rate of 25% at 10 years and more than 30% at 15 years [21]. Multifocal melanomas, extra-limbal location, incomplete surgical excision, and the lack of additional treatment are considered to be risk factors for recurrence [54, 57].

Acknowledgements

This work was supported by the College of Medicine Research Center, Deanship of Scientific Research, King Saud University, Riyadh, Saudi Arabia.

Conflict of interest

Authors do not have conflict of interest or any financial disclosures related to the above work or any of the listed items in this chapter.

Author details

Hind Alkatan* and Tariq Alzahem

*Address all correspondence to: hindkatan@yahoo.com

King Saud University, Riyadh, Kingdom of Saudi Arabia

References

[1] Chapter 1 and 2: Basic structure and function of the human cornea and adnexal structures, corneal embryology. In: Copeland and Afshari's Principles and Practice of Cornea. Vol. 1. 1st ed. New Delhi: Jaypee Brothers Medical Publishers; 2013. pp. 3-18

[2] American Academy of Ophthalmology. 2014-2015 Basic and Clinical Science Course. Section 2: Fundamentals and Principles of Ophthalmology. San Francisco, CA: American Academy of Ophthalmology; 2014. pp. 44-45

[3] American Academy of Ophthalmology. 2014-2015 Basic and Clinical Science Course. Section 8: External Disease and Cornea. San Francisco, CA: American Academy of Ophthalmology; 2014. p. 74

[4] Robertson DM, Alexander LJ, Bonanno JA, Fleiszig SMJ, McNamara N. Cornea and ocular surface disease: Application of cutting edge optometric research. Optometry and Vision Science: Official Publication of the American Academy of Optometry. 2014; **91**(401):S3-16. DOI: 10.1097/OPX.0000000000000226

[5] American Academy of Ophthalmology. 2014-2015 Basic and Clinical Science Course. Section 8: External Disease and Cornea. San Francisco, CA: American Academy of Ophthalmology; 2014. p. 9

[6] Dua HS, Faraj LA, Said DG, Gray T, Lowe J. Human corneal anatomy redefined: A novel pre-Descemet's layer (Dua's layer). Ophthalmology. 2013;**120**:1778-1785. DOI: 10.1016/j.ophtha.2013.01.018

[7] Font RL, Croxatto O, Rao N. Tumors of the Eye and Eye Adnexa. Washington: American Registry of Pathology & Armed Forces Institute of Pathology; 2006. 1-40 p

[8] Shields CL, Shields JA. Tumors of the conjunctiva and cornea. Survey of Ophthalmology. 2004;**49**:3-24. PMID: 14711437

[9] Lass JH, Jenson AB, Papale JJ, Albert DM. Papillomavirus in human conjunctival papillomas. American Journal of Ophthalmology. 1983;**95**:364-368. PMID: 6299104

[10] Lass JH, Grove AS, Papale JJ, Albert DM, Jenson AB, Lancaster WD. Detection of human papillomavirus DNA sequences in conjunctival papilloma. American Journal of Ophthalmology. 1983;**96**:670-674. PMID: 6314814

[11] Streeten BW, Carrillo R, Jamison R, Brownstein S, Font RL, Zimmerman LE. Inverted papilloma of the conjunctiva. American Journal of Ophthalmology. 1979;**88**(6):1062. PMID: 517611

[12] Shields JA, Shields CL. Eyelid, Conjunctival and Orbital Tumors. An Atlas and Textbook. 2nd ed. Philadelphia, PA: Lippincott Williams and Wilkins; 2008. pp. 250-445

[13] Jakobiec FA, Harrison W, Aronian D. Inverted mucoepidermoid papillomas of the epibulbar conjunctiva. Ophthalmology. 1987;**94**:283-287. PMID: 3587907

[14] Munro S, Brownstein S, Liddy B. Conjunctival keratoacanthoma. American Journal of Ophthalmology. 1993;**116**(5):654. PMID: 8238236

[15] Schellini SA, Marques ME, Milanezi MF, Bacchi CE. Conjunctival keratoacanthoma. Acta Ophthalmologica Scandinavica. 1997;**75**:335-337. PMID: 9253992

[16] Coupland SE, Heimann H, Kellner U, Bornfeld N, Foerster MH, Lee WR. Keratoacanthoma of the bulbar conjunctiva. The British Journal of Ophthalmology. 1998;**82**:586. PMID: 9713071

[17] Jakobiec FA, Perry HD, Harrison W, Krebs W. Dacryoadenoma. A unique tumor of the conjunctival epithelium. Ophthalmology. 1989;**96**:1014-1020. PMID: 2475840

[18] Mauriello JA Jr, Napolitano J, McLean I. Actinic keratosis and dysplasia of the conjunctiva: A clinicopathological study of 45 cases. Canadian Journal of Ophthalmology. 1995; **30**:312-316. PMID: 8574978

[19] Mittal R, Rath S, Vemuganti GK. Ocular surface squamous neoplasia-review of eti-pathogenesis and an update on clinic-pathological diagnosis. Saudi Journal of Ophthalmology. 2013;**27**:177-186. DOI: 10.1016/j.sjopt.2013.07.002

[20] Pizarello LD, Jakobeic FA. Bowens disease of the conjunctiva: A misnomer. In: Jakobeic FA, editor. Ocular and Adnexal Tumors. Birmingham, AL: Aesculapius; 1978. pp. 553-571

[21] Shields CL, Demirci H, Kara AE, Shields JA. Clinical survey of 1643 melanocytic and nonmelanocytic conjunctival tumors. Ophthalmology. 2004;**111**:1747-1754. DOI: 10.1016/j.ophtha.2004.02.013

[22] Tunc M, Char DH, Crawford B, Miller T. Intraepithelial and invasive squamous cell carcinoma of the conjunctiva: Analysis of 60 cases. The British Journal of Ophthalmology. 1999;**83**:98-103. PMID: 10209445

[23] Lee GA, Hirst LW. Ocular surface squamous neoplasia. Survey of Ophthalmology. 1995; **39**:429-450. PMID: 7660300

[24] Murthy R, Honavar SG, Vemuganti GK, Burman S, Naik M, Parathasaradhi A. Ocular surface squamous neoplasia in Papillon-Lefevre syndrome. American Journal of Ophthalmology. 2005;**139**(1):207-209. DOI: 10.1016/j.ajo.2004.07.028

[25] McKelvie PA, Daniell M, McNab A, et al. Squamous cell carcinoma of the conjunctiva: A series of 26 cases. The British Journal of Ophthalmology. 2002;**86**(2):168-173

[26] Akpek EK, Polcharoen W, Chan R, Foster CS. Ocular surface neoplasia masquerading as chronic blepharoconjunctivitis. Cornea. 1999;**18**:282-288. PMID: 10336029

[27] Tole DM, McKelvie PA, Daniell M. Reliability of impression cytology for the diagnosis of ocular surface squamous neoplasia employing the biopore membrane. The British Journal of Ophthalmology. 2001;**85**(2):154-158. PMID: 11159477

[28] Nolan GR, Hirst LW, Wright RG, et al. Application of impression cytology to the diagnosis of conjunctival neoplasms. Diagnostic Cytopathology. 1994;**11**:246-249. DOI: 10.1002/dc.2840110310

[29] Searl SS, Krigstein HJ, Albert DM, Grove AS Jr. Invasive squamous cell carcinoma with intraocular mucoepidermoid features. Conjunctival carcinoma with intraocular invasion and diphasic morphology. Archives of Ophthalmology. 1982;**100**:109-111. PMID:7055460

[30] Johnson TE, Tabbara KF, Weatherhead RG, Kersten RC, Rice C, Nasr AM. Secondary squamous cell carcinoma of the orbit. Archives of Ophthalmology. 1997;**115**:75-78. PMID: 9006429

[31] Alkatan H, Al-Motlak M, Al-Shedoukhy A. Metastatic squamous spindle cell carcinoma of the conjunctiva. Saudi Journal of Ophthalmology. 2010;**24**:155-158

[32] Asnaghi L, Alkatan H, Mahale A, et al. Identification of multiple DNA copy number alterations including frequent 8p11.22 amplification in conjunctival squamous cell carcinoma. Investigative Ophthalmology & Visual Science. 2014;**55**(12):8604-8613. DOI: 10.1167/iovs.14-14920

[33] Mahale A, Alkatan H, Alwadani S, et al. Altered gene expression in conjunctival squamous cell carcinoma. Modern Pathology. 2016;**29**(5):452-460. DOI: 10.1038/modpathol.2016.41

[34] Shields CL, Fasiuddin AF, Mashayekhi A, Shields JA. Conjunctival nevi: Clinical features and natural course in 410 consecutive patients. Archives of Ophthalmology. 2004 Feb;**122**(2):167-175. DOI: 10.1001/archopht.122.2.167

[35] Zimmerman LE, Sobin LH. International Histological Classification of Tumors. No. 24: Histological Typing of Tumors of the Eye and its Adnexa. Geneva: World Health Organization; 1980. p. 30

[36] Honavar SG, Manjandavida FP. Tumors of the ocular surface: A review. Indian Journal of Ophthalmology. 2015;**63**(3):187-203. DOI: 10.4103/0301-4738.156912

[37] To KW, Rabinowi SM, Friedman M, Cavanaugh CP. Neuro fibromatosis and neural crest neoplasms: Primary acquired melanosis and malignant melanoma of the conjunctiva. Survey of Ophthalmology. 1989;**33**:373-379. PMID: 2497540

[38] Jakobiec FA, Folberg R, Iwamoto T. Clinicopathologic characteristics of premalignant and malignant melanocytic lesions of the conjunctiva. Ophthalmology. 1989;**96**:147-166. PMID: 2649838

[39] Grossniklaus HE, Green WE, Luckenbach M, Chan CC. Conjunctival lesions in adults. A clinical and histopathologic review. Cornea. 1987;**6**(2):78-116. PMID: 3301209

[40] Paridaens AD, MacCartney AC, Hungerford JL. Multifocal amelanotic conjunctival melanoma and acquired melanin sine pigment. The British Journal of Ophthalmology. 1992;**76**(3):163-165. DOI: 10.1136/bjo.76.3.163

[41] Seregard S, Kock E. Conjunctival malignant melanoma in Sweden 1969-91. Acta Ophthalmologica, Copenhagen. 1992;**70**(3):289-296. PMID: 1636385

[42] Lommatzsch PK, Lommatzsch RE, Kirsch I, Fuhrmann P. Therapeutic outcome of patients suffering from malignant melanomas of the conjunctiva. The British Journal of Ophthalmology. 1990;**74**(10):615-619. PMID: 2285686

[43] Novais GA, Fernandes BF, Belfort RN, Castiglione E, Cheema DP, Burnier MN Jr. Incidence of melanocytic lesions of the conjunctiva in a review of 10,675 ophthalmic specimens. International Journal of Surgical Pathology. 2010;**18**(1):60-63. DOI: 10.1177/1066896908319775

[44] Norregaard JC, Gerner N, Jensen OA, Prause JU. Malignant melanoma of the conjunctiva: Occurrence and survival following surgery and radiotherapy in a Danish population. Graefe's Archive for Clinical and Experimental Ophthalmology. 1996;**234**(9):569-572. PMID: 8880155

[45] Missotten GS, Keijser S, De Keizer RJ, De Wolff-Rouendaal D. Conjunctival melanoma in the Netherlands: A nationwide study. Investigative Ophthalmology & Visual Science. 2005;**46**(1):75-82. DOI: 10.1167/iovs.04-0344

[46] Anastassiou G, Heiligenhaus A, Bechrakis N, Bader E, Bornfeld N, Steuhl KP. Prognostic value of clinical and histopathological parameters in conjunctival melanomas: A retrospective study. The British Journal of Ophthalmology. 2002;**86**(2):163-167. PMID: 11815341

[47] Shields CL, Shields JA, Gündüz K, Cater J, Market GV, Gross N, et al. Conjunctival melanoma: Risk factors for recurrence, exenteration, metastasis, and death in 150 consecutive patients. Archives of Ophthalmology. 2000;**118**(11):1497-1507. PMID: 11074806

[48] McDonnell JM, Carpenter JD, Jacobs P, Wan WL, Gilmore JE. Conjunctival melanocytic lesions in children. Ophthalmology. 1989;**96**(7):986-993. PMID: 2771364

[49] Strempel I, Kroll P. Conjunctival malignant melanoma in children. Ophthalmologica. 1999;**213**(2):129-132. PMID: 9885390

[50] Folberg R, McLean IW, Zimmerman LE. Malignant melanoma of the conjunctiva. Human Pathology. 1985;**16**(2):136-143. PMID: 3972396

[51] Jeffrey IJ, Lucas DR, McEwan C, Lee WR. Malignant melanoma of the conjunctiva. Histopathology. 1986;**10**(4):363-378

[52] Giblin ME, Shields JA, Shields CL, Eagle RC Jr. Primary eyelid malignant melanoma associated with primary conjunctival malignant melanoma. Australian and New Zealand Journal of Ophthalmology. 1988;**16**:127-131. PMID: 3179038

[53] Shields CL, Markowitz JS, Belinsky I, Schwartzstein H, George NS, Lally SE, et al. Conjunctival melanoma: Outcomes based on tumor origin in 382 consecutive cases. Ophthalmology. 2011;**118**:389-395. DOI: 10.1016/j.ophtha.2010.06.021

[54] Kenawy N, Lake SL, Coupland SE, Damato BE. Conjunctival melanoma and melanocytic intra-epithelial neoplasia. Eye. 2013;**27**(2):142-152. DOI: 10.1038/eye.2012.254

[55] Esmaeli B, Roberts D, Ross M, et al. Histologic features of conjunctival melanoma predictive of metastasis and death (an American ophthalmological thesis). Transactions of the American Ophthalmological Society. 2012;**110**:64-73. PMID: 23818735

[56] Balch CM, Wilkerson JA, Murad TM, Soong SJ, Ingalls AL, Maddox WA. The prognostic significance of ulceration of cutaneous melanoma. Cancer. 1980;**45**(12):3012-3017. PMID: 7388745

[57] Larsen AC, Dahmcke CM, Dahl C, Siersma VD, Toft PB, Coupland SE, Prause JU, Guldberg P, Heegaard S. A retrospective review of conjunctival melanoma presentation, treatment, and outcome and an investigation of features associated with BRAF mutations. JAMA Ophthalmology. 2015 Nov;**133**(11):1295-1303. DOI: 10.1001/jamaophthalmol.2015.3200

[58] Reddy HS, Keene CD, Chang SH, et al. Immunohistochemical profiling including beta-catenin in conjunctival melanocytic lesions. Experimental and Molecular Pathology. 2017;**102**(2):198-202. DOI: 10.1016/j.yexmp.2017.01.016

[59] Cao J, Brouwer NJ, Richards KE, et al. PD-L1/PD-1 expression and tumor-infiltrating lymphocytes in conjunctival melanoma. Oncotarget. 2017;**8**(33):54722-54734. DOI: 10.18632/oncotarget.18039

[60] Larsen AC, Dahl C, Dahmcke CM, Lade-Keller J, Siersma VD, Toft PB, Coupland SE, Prause JU, Guldberg P, Heegaard S. BRAF mutations in conjunctival melanoma: Investigation of incidence, clinicopathological features, prognosis and paired premalignant lesions. Acta Ophthalmologica. 2016;**94**(5):463-470. DOI: 10.1111/aos.13007

Chapter 5

Oral Cancer and Potentially Malignant Disorders

Imad Elimairi, Amel Sami and Badreldin Yousef

Additional information is available at the end of the chapter

http://dx.doi.org/10.5772/intechopen.71887

Abstract

Oral Cancer remains a greatly problematic disease with rising distribution globally, particularly the disappointing presentation among younger age groups. Varying common risk factors exist, including but not limited to premalignant disorders such as human papilloma virus (HPV) infection and immunosuppression. Genetical abnormalities and the field of epigenetics remain a new and vital piece of the puzzle in the development of Oral Cancer. Squamous cell carcinoma (SCC) remains the main histological burden with its varying counterparts; however, many types of other Oral Cancers can present in the mouth and are discussed in this chapter. More so, Oral Cancer brings with it the challenging face of diagnosis and treatment as well as effective control of metastasis. We discuss in this chapter, the epidemiology of the disease, Oral Cancer nomenclature, histological advances, clinical presentations, important risk factors, and metastatic disease pathology.

Keywords: Oral Cancer, squamous cell carcinoma, epidemiology of squamous cell carcinoma, Oral Cancer nomenclature, risk factors of squamous cell carcinoma, premalignant disorders, genetics of Oral Cancer, histological variants of squamous cell carcinoma, rare cancers of the oral cavity

1. Introduction

This chapter provides a review of Oral Cancer with a highlight of the most recent literature in its many fields. We discuss all types of Oral Cancers, but in particular SCC, the commonest type, occurring in 90–95% of Oral Cancer patients. SCC is now regarded as a neoplastic transformative process where development of malignancy is likely to occur in several stages (usually as a dysplastic lesion that progresses over time). SCC is one of the most destructive diseases in the oral cavity and thought to be the 8th most common neoplasm in the world as well as the 3rd leading cause of mortality in developing populations such as South East Asia, North Africa and Middle East and South America. The development of Oral Cancer occurs more so, among low socioeconomic groups, in males and in older populations (although SCC among younger age groups is a worrying trend, owing to HPV infection), as well as certain ethnic groups including but not limited to Africans, Americans and Caucasians who are thought to have the highest Oral Cancer rates; most likely to appear on the tongue. Asian populations tend to develop tumours in the buccal mucosa and palate. The buccal mucosa is one of the poorest prognosis sites and SCC here, is associated with rapid extension into the buccal space, metastasis and local recurrence [1]. The tongue is also an area with rapid local invasion and high recurrence risk. Certain ethnic groups also maintain genetic predispositions to Oral Cancer such as expression of N-acetyl transferase NAT1*10 genotype among the Japanese, alcohol dehydrogenase type 3 genotypes and families with history of P53 tumour suppressor gene mutations [2].

2. Oral Cancer nomenclature

Oral Cancer is often described as early or late stage disease. Early Oral Cancer exists locally, is often unilateral, has not crossed the basement membrane tissue histologically and does not include lymph node involvement. However, local disease may still be quite aggressive and require extensive reconstruction at time of surgery. Locally invasive disease refers to the spread of cells to the cervical lymph nodes. Late stage disease involves widespread or metastatic disease whereby the cancer has spread to other parts of the body. Recurrence (a tumour forming from remaining cancer cells) occurs less than 2 cm away from a previous tumour and within a duration of 3 years since treatment while a second primary disease is in relation to a new Oral Cancer development after which the primary tumour has been completely removed and thus is often more than 2 cm away from original tumour and occurs after a 3-year period [3]. However, there remain difficulties between distinguishing a recurrent lesion from a second primary tumour. Recurrence genetical diagnostics is a new field aiming to compare clones of cancer cells with previous tumour tissue within biopsy and thus the inclusion of field cancerisation concept into clinical review systems that allows better assessment of tumour risk development. Furthermore, nomenclature in regards to metastasis to lymph nodes should also be revised and can be differentiated into isolated tumour cells, micro metastasis, conventional metastasis, occult, overflow pattern, skip metastases, peppering and extracapsular spread [4].

3. Histological grading systems of Oral Cancer

TNM refers to the Tumour, Node and Metastasis staging system; a universal grading system used by clinicians worldwide. It is maintained by the Union of International Cancer Control (UICC) and the American Joint Committee on Cancer Staging (AJCC). TNM describes tumour size, spread to lymph nodes and whether there has been metastasis or not. Metastasis may further be specified according to area involved such as bone marrow (MAR), pulmonary (PUL) or osseous (OSS). T or tumour size can be classified as T0 (no primary tumour), Tis (carcinoma in situ), T1 (tumour equal or less than 2 cm), T2 (tumour equal or less than 4 cm), T3 (tumour greater than 4 cm) and T4 (tumour greater than 4 cm with deep invasion to muscle, bone or deep structures). N or lymph node involvement can be classified as N0 (no nodal involvement), N1 (ipsilateral node less than 3 cm), N2 (ipsilateral node less than 6 cm) and N3 (nodal involvement less than 6 cm or bilateral node involvement). M or Metastasis refers to M0 (no metastasis) or M1 (metastasis noted). Staging is then carried out on the background of the TNM system and aids treatment planning, maintains universal referral information and evaluates treatment. The staging system can be classified as stage 0 (carcinoma in situ), stage 1 (T1, N0, M0), stage 2 (T2, N0, M0), stage 3 (T3, N0, M0) or (T1–3, N1, M0) and stage 4 (T4, N0, M0) or (T1–4, N2, M0) or (T1–4, N1–3, M1). Finally, the grading system refers to microscopical analysis and cell differentiation histologically. This may be classified as Gx (cannot be assessed), G1 (well differentiated or low grade), G2 (moderately differentiated with elongated rete pegs invading lamina propria and keratin pearls), G3 (poorly differentiated or high grade and loss of cellular adhesion) and G4 (Undifferentiated or high grade or sheets of invading epithelium with no resemblance to normal structures). **Table 1** summaries the TNM system, staging and grading system for Oral Cancer.

Recently, it has been well established that other features in early SCC pose their own implications in tumour progression and should be paid attention to in more detail. These include depth of invasion of tumour (vertical height of tumour from level of normal epithelium) and tumour thickness (proliferative component is assessed along with vertical height).

(TNM staging system)					
Tumour size					
T0 (no primary tumour)	Tis (carcinoma in situ)	T1 (tumour equal or less than 2 cm)	T2 (tumour equal or less than 4 cm)	T3 (tumour greater than 4 cm)	T4 (tumour greater than 4 cm with deep invasion to muscle, bone, or deep structures)
Node					
	N0 (no nodal involvement),	N1 (ipsilateral node less than 3 cm)	N2 (ipsilateral node less than 6 cm)	N3 (nodal involvement less than 6 cm or bilateral node involvement).	
Metastasis					
	M0 (no metastasis)		OR	M1 (metastasis noted)	
The staging system					
	Stage 0 (carcinoma in situ)	Stage 1 (T1, N0, M0)	Stage 2 (T2, N0, M0)	Stage 3 (T3, N0, M0) or (T1–3, N1, M0)	Stage 4 (T4, N0, M0) or (T1–4, N2, M0) or (T1–4, N1–3, M1)
Grading system					
	Gx (cannot be assessed)	G1 (well differentiated)	G2 (moderately differentiated)	G3 (poorly differentiated)	G4 (undifferentiated)

Table 1. Summary of TNM staging system.

The former is now regarded as an independent factor in the TNM staging system, where the 8th edition has been modified to include: depth of invasion less than 5 cm (T1), 5–10 cm (T2) or greater than 10 cm (T3). Presence of lymphovascular and perineural invasion of tumour is associated with lymph node involvement and local recurrence. Surgical margins greater than 5 mm away from lesion are regarded as excellent, moderate if between 1 and 5 mm and poor were less than 1 mm, where the latter is associated with recurrence and poor survival rate [5]. Other histopathological predictors include sialadenotropism, involvement of underlying skin and the histological variant of the SCC.

Other types of grading systems include the WHO (International agency on Cancer) grading system, based on labelling tumours as well, moderately or poorly differentiated. However, the WHO itself states this system has its limitations on prognosis of Oral Cancer but could be improved when margins are analysed. Broder's classification breaks down tumours into four different grades according to degree of differentiation and keratinisation of tumour cells; Anneroth's grading considers keratinisation, nuclear polymorphism, the number of mitoses, the pattern and stage of invasion and lymphoplasmacytic infiltration within thickness of tumour and Bryne's grading is based on assessing the invasive front excluding mitotic count [6].

The type of invasion front has also been described where 4 patterns may be noted histologically. These include type 1 or tumour with a cohesive advancing front, type 2 or incohesive front with malignant keratinocytes distributed as islands or sheets penetrating at different levels, type 3 or dyscohesion with budded tiny islands of cells at the advancing front and type 4 or super non-cohesion where by malignant keratinocytes invade as individual units [4].

4. Predisposing risk factors for the development of Oral Cancer

The pathogenesis of Oral Cancer is multifactorial. Genetic damage, microorganisms and carcinogens such as tobacco and alcohol are just some of the major risk factors that predispose to Oral Cancer. Tumour microenvironment such as vascular network proximity to tumour, glucose and lactate concentrations, interstitial fluid pressure, PH extracellularity [7] and interconnections between non-cancer cells and cancer cells all have important associations with Oral Cancer development. Furthermore, hypoxia plays an important role in cancer cell progression, whereby rapid growth of cancer cells leads to a hypoxic environment particularly at the centre of SCC lesions, further increasing their proliferative capacity and malignancy capability. Under these hypoxic conditions, cells undergo the 'Epithelial Mesenchymal Transition (EMT)' where epithelial cells become more fibroblastic in nature and thus more invasive with metastatic potential [6, 8]. The presence of fibroblasts in the environment further leads to growth of epithelial cells with assisted keratinocyte growth factor stimulation. EMT leads to cancer cell movement, ease of invasion and metastasis. Cancer stem cells which are either derived from adult stem cells, the possible fusion of haematogenic stem cells with a differentiated epithelial cell or neosis, have the ability to self-propagate, give rise to different tumour cell populations and allow their differentiation.

It has been postulated that these cancer stem cells have a distinctive phenotype, allowing them to initiate growth of a tumour, control the lineage of tumour growth pattern as well as have lasting power that supports their transformation into malignancy and sustainability through cell mutations. Field cancerisation is a concept implicated in the development of multiple primary tumours, recurrence and second primary tumours. Patients with previous history of SCC in particular or upper aero-digestive tract neoplasms are thought to be at risk up to 35% for the development of another tumour and the prognosis is often poorer for this presenting lesion. Pre-neoplastic alterations, particularly genetic, are thought to lead to field cancerisation. Where cell lines are monoclonal (same mutated lineage of cells), field cancerisation may occur through the process of exportation of cells to adjacent mucosa or through saliva. Where there is polyclonal tumorisation (different mutated lineages of cells), field cancerisation is thought to occur due to the whole cavity being exposed to carcinogens and susceptibility to genetic alterations [3]. Sustainment of angiogenesis is another primary factor in the progression of Oral Cancer where nutrients are provided as well as provision of routes for the development of the tumour away from the primary site and penetration of the circulatory system.

4.1. Potentially malignant disorders

In 2005, the WHO advised to merge both the terms 'potentially malignant lesions' and 'potentially malignant conditions' and classify all these disorders as 'potentially malignant disorders' [9]. Detection of potentially malignant disorders may go unnoticed due to their painless nature. These include White Leukoplakic (Homogenous), Mixed (non-homogenous or speckled) and Red Erythroplakic lesions. Others include actinic cheilitis, lichen planus and submucous fibrosis and systemic/discoid lupus erythromatosis as well as rarer conditions that include dyskeratosis congenita (predisposition to leukoplakic lesions), Plummer–Vinson syndrome, Fanconi's anaemia, Epidermolysis bullosa dystrophicans and Xeroderma Pigmentosum. Chronic Immunosuppression is also a risk factor in the development of Oral Cancer.

Dysplasia is described by the WHO as either mild, moderate or severe, and can present in any such form in potentially malignant disorders. New literature also suggests the term 'oral intraepithelial neoplasia' rather than the term 'dysplasia' be used which describes better the histological picture. This includes epithelial proliferation that can be papillary or verrucous, drop-shaped rete ridges, skip areas of normal mucosa where dysplastic epithelium can be found, and hyperorthokeratosis as well as cellular changes including nuclear hyperchromatism, pleomorphism, altered nuclear/cytoplasmic ratio, excess mitotic activity, loss of polarity of cells, loss of differentiation, loss of intercellular adherence and deep cell keratinisation. However, the histological grading of dysplastic lesions is not an accurate method to conclude which lesions are in danger of becoming an SCC as there is a high degree of subjectivity from pathological observers and recent evidence suggests there is little or no correlation between dysplastic grade and progressions to Oral Cancer [10]. Recent studies highlight that variations in length between the apical membrane of basal cells and the basement membrane as well as the disordered arrangement of these cells may be useful in the study of dysplastic lesions [11]. Several biomarkers have been studied to assess the prognosis of dysplastic lesions, other than histopathological picture and include S100A7, DNA content, DNA ploidy, loss of heterozygosity, p16 methylation, hypermethylation of endothelin receptor type b, kinesin family member 1A [12], the assessment of proliferation marker Ki-67 and cytokeratins 13 and 17 which have all been implicated in the development of SCC from a dysplastic lesion.

4.1.1. Leukoplakias

Leukoplakia is defined as 'a white patch or plaque that cannot be scraped off and cannot be clinically or histopathologically determined as any other disease'. Histopathologically, Leukoplakias represent a wide spectrum of non-specific epithelial changes ranging from hyperkeratosis that overlies a thickened acanthotic but ordered mucosa to lesions with marked dysplasia or even carcinoma in situ upon biopsy. The Leukoplakic clinical picture ranges from a thin smooth homogenous white appearance to increased fissuring or a lesion that is verrucous and nodular in nature. The non-homogenous Leukoplakia and Erythroplakia are the most likely to have severe dysplasia or carcinoma in situ, where the latter is of a red appearance due to superficial erosion and an intense inflammatory reaction with vascular dilatation. 'Proliferative Multifocal Leukoplakia (PML)' is a new term to describe verrucous leukoplakia and its concurrent risk for development into verrucous SCC carcinoma, with more accuracy, so that clinicians are aware that in its initial stages even if it is not so verrucous in appearance clinically, there may be frank carcinoma evident histopathologically. PML also has a high rate of Cancerous progression in relation to anatomical location (soft and hard palate, alveolar ridge, buccal and labial mucosa, attached gingivae and gingival sulcus and floor of mouth), gender (more in women) and in those who do not possess risk factors such as smoking and alcohol [13]. It is thought only 1–5% of Leukoplakias progress to cancer; however, there is still no robust method of identifying those lesions that will or will not do so. Subsequently, there is wide variation in the treatment of Leukoplakia among clinicians, whereby some clinicians choose to monitor (except severe dysplasia where excision must occur) and others prefer to remove lesions regardless of histological pattern.

4.1.2. Lichen planus

A T-cell mediated disease with tumour necrosis factor-alpha (TNF-alpha) drive, Lichen planus presents clinically as either reticular, annular, plaque-like, atrophic or erosive forms. About 1–5% of lesions of Lichen planus may develop malignant SCC change [14], but the risk is low. Histologically, the term lichenoid dysplasia is a picture of band-like lymphocytic infiltrate underneath dysplastic epithelium that may have an increased risk of malignant change.

4.1.3. Oral submucous fibrosis

This premalignant condition is mainly restricted to Asian populations who use betel quid and areca. Progressive irreversible fibrosis and hyalinisation initiates in the lamina propria with progressive destruction of connective tissue, muscle and fat as well as atrophy of overlying epithelium and change of the normal colour of the mucosa to white/grey. Trismus is a final stage manifestation that may be so severe (due to the formation of fibrous bands in the cheeks, around the lips and fauces) that SCC discovery may be hindered [9].

4.1.4. Actinic cheilitis

Ranging histologically from hyperkeratosis to SCC in situ, actinic cheilitis is a clinical term for a white, ulcerative crusted lesion to the vermillion border of the lips, which is mainly present in older men due to sun exposure.

4.2. Immunological and genetical basis of Oral Cancer

The immune system plays a vital role in either the eradication of malignant cells or their promotion into a neoplasm. Monocytes and macrophages may play a role against tumour progression by releasing proinflammatory cytokines such as Il-2, TNF-alpha and reactive nitrogen particles that exhibit cytotoxic and cytostatic activity as well as promoting dendritic and natural killer cells in the location as a response against cancer cells or on the contrary; the monocyte/macrophage system may be induced to promote neoplastic change by aiding the expression of angiopoietin 2, vascular endothelial growth factor A, chemokine ligand 3 and adhesion molecules that are key in tumour progression [15]. Unlike some genetic disorders which have a distinct development of cancers associated with them such as Multiple Endocrine Neoplasia 2, Fanconi's anaemia, Bloom syndrome, Gorlin Goltz syndrome, Peutz Jeghers syndrome, Li Fraumeni syndrome, Xeroderma pigmentosum and Familial Retinoblastoma [16], Oral Cancer has not been implicated yet with a specific genetic disorder or genetic polymorphism, rather its formation is due to a combination of mutations and progression of damaged cells into cancer sustainability.

Chromosomal alterations and/or epigenetic alterations occur in both premalignant lesions and SCC, and new diagnostic mechanisms as well as therapeutics often target this area. Genomic instability of Oral Cancer involves defects in DNA damage repair, loss of heterozygosity such as that of 9q33 present in nearly 30% of SCC lesions and of 9p21 associated with loss of tumour suppressor activity, defects in chromosomal segregation which are thought to promote resistance against treatment within cancer cells, copy number alterations, loss of telomere stability which leads to prevention of cell destruction and is highly expressed in SCC cells, and regulation of DNA checkpoints. An SCC develops when such genetic changes and others are not counterbalanced, leading to a combination of activation of proto-oncogenes, deactivation of growth inhibitory pathways and loss of function of tumour suppressor genes. Epigenetics deals in particular with defects such as DNA methylation, histone modifications and RNA-mediated silencing. Furthermore, some genetical alterations occur in particular locations of the SCC such as at the invasive front where heterozygosity and microsatellite instability at chromosomal loci TP53 and RPS6 occur more so than in its central or superficial portions [6]. Other genetic defects involved in Oral Cancer include disruption to apoptosis such as CASP8 mutations which inhibit extrinsic apoptotic pathways, immortalisations, and signal transducers, improvement of angiogenesis and gain of growth factor receptors, such as epidermal growth factor receptor (EGFR) [17].

Three distinct regions of deletions have been identified in chromosome 3p associated with development of Oral Cancer [18]. Promoter hypermethylation results in inactivation of the p16 gene, which is an inhibitor of cyclin dependant kinase family of serine/threonine kinases on chromosome 11q13 that activates cell cycle progression and promotes dysplastic cell tissue invasion leading to normal epithelium becoming hyperplastic/hyperkeratotic epithelium. 5-hydroxymethylcytosine, found more in well-differentiated cells, is reduced in dysplastic lesions and SCC and may be associated with the stage of differentiation of malignant cells [19]. The further loss of heterozygosity at 17p with point mutations in the p53 tumour suppression gene leads to cell dysplasia. Genomic alterations to 4q, 6p, 8p, 11q, 13q and 14q have all been implicated in the development of malignant changes.

MicroRNAs (MiRs) are small non-coding RNAs that regulate transcription and may act as either oncogenes (where their overexpression promotes cancerous changes), or as tumour suppressor genes (where their under expression leads to tumorogenesis). MiR7, MiR-21, MiR-24 and MiR-184 when upregulated are implicated in the development of premalignant lesions and the development of SCC while the downregulation of MiR-375 can lead to tumorogenesis via inability to inhibit migration of cancer cells, CAL27 cells. Those lesions with higher expressions of MiR-375 have a protective factor against SCC development [20]. Other downregulated tumour suppressor MiRs includes MiR-133a & b (where their loss un-inhibits the expression of oncogene PKM2), MiR 26a-5p (prevents proliferation of cells, cell cycle progression and induces apoptosis of CAL27 cells) and MiR 34a-5p (its downregulation allows for uncontrolled progression of CAL27 and SCC-15 cells) as well as others such as MiR-29b, MiR-138, MiR-182, MiR-195, MiR-205 and MiR-219, whereby their loss leads to overexpression of oncogenic factors such as G protein alpha inhibiting activity polypeptide 2, Insulin Growth Factor 1 Receptor, Protein Kinase C1 and Survivin [21]. Survivin, an inhibitor of apoptosis, may also be activated by HPV E26 protein when there is reduced expression of p53 and leads to aggressive tumour formation and resistance to treatment, not only in Oral Cancer but also among several other systemic cancers such as breast, thyroid, colorectal, medulloblastoma and glioblastomas [22].

Upregulation of NOTCH 1 expression between cells can act as an oncogene or tumour suppressor gene, stimulating progenitor cells in SCC of the head and neck. The Dachshund homologue 1 is also a tumour suppressor gene where its expression can prevent migration and adhesion of cancer cells and can target cancer cell lines, such as SCC—25 cells, thus functioning as a growth inhibitor [23]. However, its frequent methylation in Oral Cancer leads to its reduced expression and it has been associated with poorly differentiated tumours and lymph node metastasis, in particular SCC affecting the tongue.

EGFR is a proto-oncogene and a tyrosine kinase-based receptor, known to be overexpressed in many systemic cancers such as breast, non-small cell lung cancer and colorectal cancer and leads to uncontrolled cell division. The overexpression of subtype epidermal growth factor (EGF) 4 has been associated with lymph node metastasis in SCC in the oral cavity. Indeed, therapeutics that target subtypes 1 to 4 EGF include cetuximab (reported rarely in treatment of SCC) and trastuzumab, MM-121, AM, G888, TK-A3 and TK-A4 which have been used clinically for other cancer treatments but not for SCC [24]. Argyrophilic nucleolar organising regions (ribosomal DNA) are located on the short arm of chromosome 13, 14, 15, 21 and 22 and when assessed through silver staining techniques, they can be correlated with cellular proliferation of Oral Cancer. Abnormal chromosomal segregation or DNA mono or aneuploidy is also a marker for Cancer formation; however, this remains controversial [25].

4.3. Other markers

Vascular endothelial growth factor C and its receptors such as Flt-4 (class 3 tyrosine receptor kinases) may be released not only by the primary tumour as oncogenes but also by macrophages and surrounding vascular endothelial cells and have a strong role to play in the transmission of metastasis to lymph nodes. Tumour lymphangiogenesis is thought to be promoted by VEGF C expression, particularly in early stages [26, 27]. Transforming growth factor B1 may have tumour suppressor activity in the early stages of Oral Cancer, although it has been widely implicated in the progression of the disease (in particular secondary tumours) by aiding the proliferation of tumour SCC cell lines and their survival, allowing the activation of p63 on chromosome 3 and C-Myc oncogene that leads to cell proliferation and transcription and inhibition of E Cadherin repressors, thus allowing for EMT, an important factor in the progression of SCC [28].

Toll-like receptor (TLR)-4 is expressed by cancer cells, allowing for protection from the immune system and resistance of cancer cells against apoptosis as well as promoting cancer progression, cancer growth, invasion and metastasis. The TLRs further activate protein signalling group NF-kb, in particular nuclear p65, which is important in the progression of malignancy states by inhibiting apoptotic mechanisms. SCC patients with high TLR-4 expression were found to have more aggressive disease and poorer prognosis. Some new therapeutics such as TAK-242 and Eps 7630 working against TLRs specifically and NF kb respectively and some have been trialled in SCC therapy [29].

Proteolysis (degradation of basement membrane by enzymes) occurs in particular by matrix metalloproteinase (MMPS) expression and has an important role to play in the progression of cancer cells. MMP2 has been shown to digest type 3 collagen and disrupt the basement membrane as well as degrading other extracellular matrix proteins [30]. E Cadherins are cell-cell adhesion molecules where their low expression is related to poorly differentiated tumours and metastatic ability. Increased expression of EpCam adhesion molecules further down-regulates Cadherin adhesion and promotes segregation of tumour cells and their metastasis [31].

4.4. Tobacco

Tobacco has been used for centuries and is a well-known carcinogenic material leading to the promotion of all types of bodily cancers; not exclusive to Oral Cancer development alone. Tobacco can come in the form of cigarettes, (both classic and electronic), cigar, pipe, reverse smoking, and as smokeless tobacco. 75% of people with Oral Cancer smoke [32] and the use of smokeless tobacco provides a unique trouble to the oral cavity whereby products are placed directly on oral tissues with increased concentration of nitrosamines absorbed both locally and systemically. Examples of smokeless tobacco products from around the world include Betel quid and Paan in Asia, Shammah in Saudi Arabia, Khat in Yemen and Toombak in Sudan. Tobacco involves a dose response relationship whereby the level of exposure (increased time, quantity and concentration) determines the risk of developing a tobacco-related dysplasia and tobacco-related Oral Cancer. When cessation arises, the risk of developing Oral Cancer presumes normality after 10–15 years of abstinence. The use of electronic cigarettes is a new area, where the true risk of Oral Cancer development and formation of premalignant lesions in those using electronic cigarettes is yet to be elucidated in Long–term research follow-ups. More younger people are now using electronic cigarettes but their nicotine levels may be higher than what manufacturers advertise. Electronic cigarettes and the heating of E liquids to high temperatures may also release other carcinogenic compounds such as carbonyl compounds (formaldehyde, acetaldehyde and acrolein) that may be SCC associated. Nicotine replacement therapy has also been implicated as a potential factor for SCC development.

4.5. Alcohol

Ethanol is both a topical and systemic carcinogen and its metabolite acetaldehyde is an even more potent one. Local contact leads to direct irritation of tissues and is thought to promote direct carcinogenic change. The metabolisation of ethanol to acetaldehyde is carried out by alcohol dehydrogenase. Acetaldehyde is cytotoxic and leads to production of free radicals as well as activating N Nitrosamines by inducing the CYP1A1 cascade [2]. The use of alcohol and tobacco together leads to a potent synergistic affect (almost a 30 times higher risk of developing SCC when compared to non-users) and is implicated widely in SCC development. Alcohol here, may act as a solvent for carcinogens within tobacco smoke. Finally, the presence of alcohol in mouthwashes, around 20%, and its role in causing Oral Cancer has also been a point of highlight. No strong evidence exists to conclude that the presence of alcohol among these products is significantly responsible for carcinomatous change, as well as the fact that those patients who did develop Oral Cancer while using alcohol mouthwashes also had confounding factors, especially the use of tobacco. However, a large retrospective study on 8981 cases of Head and Neck SCC by the International Head and Neck Cancer Epidemiology Consortium suggested that heavy frequent and long-term users of alcoholic mouthwashes as well as persons with poor oral hygiene or those who replace oral hygiene with use of mouthwash may have a significant connection [33].

4.6. Infections

4.6.1. Human papilloma viruses (HPVs)

18–72% of oropharyngeal SCC (tonsils, oropharynx and base of tongue) harbour oncogenic HPV proteins that helps to induce DNA damage, cell cycle dysregulation and keratinocyte dysregulation, but the exact method of how HPV initiates and maintains the development of SCC is still not completely known. The tumour suppressor genes p53 (Arg72pro) and pRb are inactivated by E6 and E7 viral oncoproteins respectively but not all oropharyngeal tumours are E6/E7 positive [34]. The most common HPV infection is HPV 16, but 18, 31, 33, and 35 are also implicated in SCC development. HPV positive SCCs are often non-keratinising with ovoid cells, indistinct cytoplasm and contain other distinct histological features namely mitosoid cells or nuclear fragmentation, presence of apoptotic and dyskeratotic cells with hyperchromatin and cytoplasmic eosinophilia [35]. The role of HPV infection and SCC of the anterior tongue is also a target for further studies. Several HPVs, particularly the recent HPV 56, has also been implicated in SCC of the anterior tongue with poorer outcomes [36].

While it has been generally accepted that patients with positive HPVSCC have an improved prognosis compared to those with negative HPVSCC, this statement is subject to debate. HPV positivity is thought to increase sensitivity to treatments and apoptotic induction as well triggering of the immune response to clear damaged cells. However, some studies have recently suggested a poor prognosis for positive HPVSCC due to HPV positive cells stimulating lymphocyte production and promoting cytokines with an immune profile that promotes HPV infected cancer cell replication. Furthermore, it has been analysed that predictivity of improved outcome is related to other factors such as viral load and transcriptional activity rather than just presence or absence of virus. High viral load with increased E6/E7 expression and transcriptional activity, improves prognosis outcome as these tumours have a distinct phenotype of less chromosomal abnormalities compared to low viral load associated tumours. Vaccines Cervarix and Gardasil are given to adolescent women to protect against cervical cancer but their role in preventing Oral Cancer in both females and males is still under promising research.

4.6.2. Epstein-Barr virus (EBV)

Non-keratinising forms of nasopharyngeal carcinoma are implicated by EBV infection. EBVs are also well known in the association of B-cell lymphomas (in particular Burkitt's Lymphoma), anaplastic carcinoma, salivary gland tumours, but recent literature examines its possible role in the initiation and progression of Oral Cancer SCC. Dysplastic changes among epithelial cells renders them more likely to express CD21, allowing the abundant glycoprotein gp350 of EBV to bind to plasma membrane easily and give it an entry into epithelial cells. An increase in CK19 expression is then observed where the former is a possible stem cell marker and has been associated with premalignant changes and poorly differentiated SCC development. EBV-infected epithelial tissues have been shown to express higher CK19 compared to healthy controls [37]. Furthermore, infection by EBV may allow a growth advantage of mutant cells whereby EBV proteins and transcripts may alter cell behaviour by increasing their proliferation rate. EBV has also been found within keratin pearls and within malignant epithelial cells [38].

4.6.3. Candidiasis

Although controversial, harbouring candida (C) infections has been associated with the development of SCC. However, because these fungi remain a part of normal oral flora, the carcinogenic ability of C infection in some patients remain unclear. Mutagenic C strains, presence of chronic inflammation, production of carcinogens such as nitrosamines by the fungi, their ability to metabolise procarcinogens, and secretion of proteolytic enzymes that damage basement membrane (loss of laminin 332 and E-Cadherins important in keratinocyte adhesion) remain key factors. Recent studies have established SCC development to increased fungi carriage in patients with both dysplasia and SCC compared to healthy controls. *C. albicans* produces a local environment that favours cell proliferation and tumour cell expansion. Furthermore, patients with chronic C infection have been found to have increased salivary IL-10, associated with poor SCC prognosis. IL-10 although has the beneficial role of balancing the inflammatory environment, leads to neoplastic succession by inactivating the innate immune system [39]. *C. albicans* also induce IL-8 secretion, stimulating the production of TNF-alpha; a potent inflammatory mediator possible aggravating local tissues and thus help drive formation of SCC. NFkb is an important cancer promoter that is induced when *C. albicans* activates TLRs that interact with NFkb and the production of chronic inflammatory mediators all leading to a cancer pro-environment [40].

C. albicans genotypes are thought to differ in patients who develop SCC (*C. albicans* genotype A) compared to healthy controls (*C. albicans* genotype B) where these different strains may have increased carcinogenic potential. Also, *C. albicans* converts ethanol to the carcinogenic metabolite acetaldehyde as well as hydroxyethyl radicals, ethoxy radicals and hydroxy radicals which can all potentiate SCC development when alcohol is chronically consumed [41]. Patients with Chronic hyperplastic candidiasis (CHC), for example, are well known to have increased malignant transformation most likely due to the release of the potent carcinogen, N-nitrosobenzylmethylamine formation that leads to keratinocyte cell aggravation. Treatment with triazoles and cessation of smoking may resolve some lesions although this is not definite in all cases. *C. albicans* study from CHC biopsy samples were found to have increased Adh1p m RNA expression, an isoenzyme that majorly catalyses ethanol into acetaldehyde thus potentiating carcinogenesis in these lesions [40].

4.6.4. Bacterial pathogens

Chronic inflammation aids progression of SCC development by increasing malignant cell proliferation, cell survival, stimulation of neoangiogenesis and reducing anti-tumour immunity. Although small, a significant connection between presence of periodontal disease, an important and common type of local chronic inflammation in the oral cavity and development of Oral Cancer may exist. Periodontal disease offers a proinflammatory environment with a display of varying polymorphonuclear cells, presence of proinflammatory local and systemic cytokines (TNF-alpha, Il-6, C-reactive protein), proinflammatory proteins (MMPs) and proangiogenic factors, all aiding neoplastic promotion. Chronic inflammation is further advanced by microbial toxins and bacteria associated with periodontal disease (*Streptococcus sanguis, Prevotella melaninogenica, S. mitis* others) that may have a role in causing disruption to normal cell growth and prospective tumour formation [42]. Periodontal pathogens have also been associated with promoting EMT in SCC [43], an important factor in progression to metastasis. Furthermore, the periodontal pathogens, *Porphyromonas gingivalis* and *Fusobacterium nucleatum,* may increase SCC invasion and aggressiveness. These bacteria may also contribute to cancer development by activating tumour signalling pathways Nfkb and STAT3 leading to production of anti-apoptotic proteins and release of growth factors such as EGF, TNF-alpha and transforming growth factor, and all SCC promoters [44]. HPV E6/E6 mRNA in one study was detected in periodontal pockets and gingival sulcus, a possible risk factor for aiding viral-associated Oral Cancer development.

http://dx.doi.org/10.5772/intechopen.71887

4.6.5. Syphilis

Although syphilitic leukoplakia and its development into SCC is generally a historic finding, an association between tertiary syphilis and development of Oral Cancer, is still being reported. Cases with overriding SCC on syphilitic gumma as well as several reports of syphilitic patients developing Kaposi's sarcoma are present in the current literature. However, direct scientific association has not yet been studied and other risk factors such as these patients also using tobacco and alcohol, being malnourished and being co-infected with HIV, generally confuse the true link between syphilis and development of Oral Cancer. Nevertheless, this relationship cannot be completely neglected and thus should be given some credibility in clinical practice in order to determine those patients with Oral Cancer who do turn out to present with undiagnosed or late-stage syphilitic disease [45, 46].

5. Dietary factors

Antioxidants such as Vitamin A, C and E and other trace elements have a protective role against development of SCC and thus when deficient have been associated with SCC in the oral cavity and other organs. Interestingly, people with a high intake of meat and processed meat products are at higher risk of developing Oral Cancer. Iron deficiency is well known to cause epithelial atrophy and patients with post-cricoid web (Plummer Vinson/Patterson-Kelly syndrome) have an increased risk of developing Oral Cancer.

6. Radiation

6.1. Ultraviolet

Although skin cancers are more associated with sun exposure, persons whom are highly sensitive to UV exposure such as those who are fair skinned, with solid organ transplantation (particularly an association between kidney transplants and lower lip cancer), as well as with the autosomal recessive condition Xeroderma pigmentosum have an increased predisposition to development of SCC. Women are thought to be better protected from sun-exposed lip cancer due to the use of lipstick. Patients with occupational hazards such as fishermen and farmers and other sun-exposed workers have an increased risk of lower lip cancer. Cases of lower lip cancer in those with renal transplants are unique in particular [47] in that cancer is often preceded by actinic keratosis and dysplasia and worryingly, tumours are often quite subtle in appearance [48] with a short clinical presentation time. It is thought that UV-B radiation enhances immunosuppression locally and impairs antigen presenting Langerhans cells that help eradicate cancer cells.

6.2. Therapeutic

Ionising radiation for the treatment of head and neck cancers poses a problematic risk factor for the development of new primary oral malignancies, most commonly aggressive sarcomas and salivary gland tumours. The dose of radiation, exposure time and other factors play a role in the development of such lesions. However, radiation exposure may also have a beneficial effect (see Section 9) in protection against SCC development.

7. Immunosuppression

Patients on long-term immunosuppressive medications such as Cyclosporine and Azathioprine as well as other immunosuppressive drugs following transplantations are more at risk of developing Oral Cancer. These drugs are known to lead to DNA mutations, possibly within keratinocytes. Patients with kidney and liver transplants have been shown to develop lip cancer in particular as well as chronic graft versus host disease patients. Patients with Crohns disease who are on long-term azathioprine have also been reported to have an increased risk of developing tongue cancer. Another important factor is the possible HLA incompatibility that arises between host and recipient that triggers the host's immune system and leads to the potentiation of neoplastic progression of cells [49]. HIV infection is another factor where the disease predisposes its patients to increased development of Kaposi's sarcoma and lymphomas (plasmablastic) that may present in the oral cavity; however, the development of Oral Cancer SCC in HIV patients is more likely to be in relation to secondary HPV infection, or Tobacco use.

8. Dental implants

Recent reports highlight a possible link with placement of dental implants and SCC. It is thought that implants may act as a traumatic or irritating factor and SCC has been reported in the peri-implantary tissues in about 1.5% of SCC patients [50]. Peri-implantary inflammation can lead to a persistent promotion of cellular proliferation and cell survival and even the activation of oncogenes and inactivation of tumour suppressor genes. Furthermore, titanium material may not be as inert as originally thought bringing about an allergic reaction and an inflammatory background to tissues. Where there is implant looseness, further activation of inflammation (predisposing factor to SCC) may occur. Implants coated with hydroxyapatite may induce a mucositis with reports of SCC developing 1-year post implantation. Some cases of metastasis (breast, lung and prostate) around implants have also been described in the literature and may be up to 1%. Patients who undergo radiation with implants in place may be subjected to dispersion of the radiation produced, where the dose is increased in front of the implant and decreased posteriorly allowing theoretically for SCC recurrence as well as the possibility of migration of malignant cells through the peri-implantary sulcus to the jaws. Finally, corrosion products such as titanium dioxide may have carcinogenic potential and metallic ions from implants may act as immunodepressants or create a cytotoxic environment [51]. **Table 2** summaries the predisposing risk factors for the development of Oral Cancer.

http://dx.doi.org/10.5772/intechopen.71887

Predisposing risk factors for the development of Oral Cancer					
Local factors	**Potentially malignant disorders**	**Genetical abnormalities**	**Use of tobacco**	**Infections that may predispose to development of Oral Cancer**	**Other factors**
• Vascular network proximity • Low glucose levels • High lactate concentrations • High interstitial fluid pressure • Hypoxic environment and • Development of epithelial mesenchymal transition	• White • Mixed leukoplakic • Red Erythroplakic lesions • Actinic cheilitis • Lichen planus • Submucous fibrosis • Systemic/ Discoid Lupus Erythromatosis • Dyskeratosis congenita • Others	• Chromosomal alterations (segregation, telomere instability, copy number alterations) • Epigenetic changes (DNA methylation, histone modification, RNA mediated silencing) • DNA damage repair • Loss of heterozygosity Genetical causations for Oral Cancer	• Cigarette • Electronic • Cigar • Pipe • Reverse smoking • Smokeless tobacco Use of alcohol • Ethanol • Ethanol by-products (acetaldehyde) • Nitrosamine contaminants	• Human papilloma virus • Epstein Barr virus • Candidiasis • Bacterial pathogens • Syphilis	• Dietary factors (low anti-oxidants, iron deficiency, and malnutrition) • -Immunosuppression HIV infection persons on Immunosuppressive medications i.e. transplant patients
Local concepts • Field cancerisation • Sustained angiogenesis Others • Radiation exposure • Dental Implants		• Activation of protooncogenes • Loss of tumour suppressor genes • Disruption of apoptosis	Combined tobacco and alcohol use • Synergistic compounded increased Oral Cancer predisposition		

Table 2. Predisposing factors.

9. Factors that may reduce the risk of development of Oral Cancer

Antioxidants are needed for normal growth and differentiation of epithelial tissues where deficiencies can lead to the replacement of metastatic squamous epithelium. Vitamins A, C and E have a protective effect against the induction of tumour formation and their presence and strengthens resistance against tumour formation. A recent study [52] suggests that phenolic compounds such as caffeic and coumaric acids may have a protective role against the development of Oral Cancer. These compounds may prevent oxidative DNA damage. Caffeine has even been proven to reverse cell cycle and have a role in the apoptotic pathway. A meta-analysis on tea consumption highlights a protective effect, particularly from green tea, due to its ability from theaflavins and catechins to induce apoptosis and inhibit cancer cell growth [53]. Radiation therapy has also been shown to have a beneficial effect in reducing the development of second primary tumours, whereby adjacent mucosa that may already have had premalignant changes after irradiation is prevented from further malignant transformation [54, 55].

10. Detection of Oral Cancer

Early detection is vital in improving the prognosis of Oral Cancer and can minimise adverse effects of treatment such as surgery reconstruction and help maintain quality of life. Practitioners may have a role to play in the Misdiagnosis, Mistreatment, and Mismanagement of SCC particularly in regards to dysplastic lesions. In general, a lesion that cannot be wiped off and persists for more than 3 weeks should be regarded as highly suspicious unless proven otherwise by trustworthy means. It is important not to forget histological resemblance of well-differentiated squamous cell carcinoma to benign epithelial proliferation, seen adjacent to chronic ulcers and infections, thus Oral Cancer may have several differential diagnoses [56]. As a clinician, one cannot underestimate diligent history taking, visual inspection and digital examination in the early diagnosing of Oral Cancer. When Oral Cancer is detected, all patients must undergo full clinical investigations of the body such as blood pressure, heart, liver and renal function (urea and electrolytes), haematological picture, blood group and calcium levels. Locally, histopathological examination remains the mainstay form of investigation. Early tumours often have no local or distant spread and the 5-year survival for early stage detection is 80% compared to 19% when late finding occurs [57]. Several mainstay and new mechanisms in the detection of Oral Cancer are highlighted below.

10.1. Toluidine blue

Toluidine blue is used to optimally select a biopsy site and also aids in the assessment of lesion margins during surgery. The product binds to DNA (mitochondrial, altered and increased DNA) and thus is a vital stain that is not precancer or cancer specific (can also stain traumatic lesions and non-cancerous ulceration) but does have great sensitivity for dysplastic and cancerous lesions. Some studies have shown a positive correlation with toluidine blue and lesions with loss of heterozygosity. The latter information provides further evidence that toluidine blue may have advantage in detecting seemingly sound lesions that may have pre-cancerous non-visible molecular changes. Strength of stain colour should not be regarded of phenotypical importance as both weak and strong staining of an area suggest suspicious molecular profiles [10, 58].

10.1.1. *Iodine solutions*

Iodine solutions such as Lugol's iodine and dental iodine glycerine may be used to detect dysplastic and/or cancerous lesions. Iodine binds to glycogen in the normal epithelium creating a brown/black stain but diseased lesions do not stain effectively. It may be particularly useful in the delineation of lesion margins where they become more sharply defined [59].

10.1.2. *Light detection*

Cancer cells are thought to refract and absorb light differently due to their structural and metabolic differences compared to healthy cells calling for the field of light detection-based systems in diagnosing Oral Cancer. These include chemiluminescence or Vizilite (normal epithelium appears blue-white, while abnormal appears distinctly white), Vizilite plus which contains pre-toluidine blue use, tissue luorescence or Veloscope that aims to detect loss of fluorescence in lesions that are dysplastic or malignant, and tissue fluorescence spectroscopy. These aids are useful adjuncts to diagnosis and therapy, whereby they can obtain safer margins during surgery; however, generally they are not as effective in distinguishing between high-risk and low-risk premalignant lesions [57]. Other weaknesses of these systems include low specificity, high cost and limited sturdy evidence regards their reproducibility and reliability [10].

10.1.3. *Laser*

Matrix-assisted laser desorption spectrometry and ionisation of serum may prove beneficial in the detection of proteins by assessing their hydrophobic and hydrophilic anionic and cationic metal-binding properties. These proteins include C terminal fragments of the fibrinogen alpha chain and is highly specific and sensitive for cancer presence [60]. Laser scanning confocal microscopy is a new tool that can detect dysplastic changes after application of a fluorescent cellular contrast (acriflavine hydrochloride) and gives rise to optical sections that are visualised digitally through a live stream image. Cellular structures are highlighted in more precise detail; the multiple cell layers of the oral epithelium (from the surface to basal layer) are analysed for morphological characteristics; polymorphisms in size and shape of cells are much clearer; and dysplastic cell location can be accurately determined. Digital laser technology, thus, is a form of diagnosis that can provide the opportunity for a new histological era… 'the digital histologist' [57].

10.1.4. *Exfoliative cytology*

Cells on the surface of dysplasia/carcinoma can be assessed and is termed 'Exfoliative cytology'. This method can be used in screening a wide number of people/populations as well as serving as an aid in guiding optimum biopsy taking, but may overestimate dysplastic lesions and thus produce false positive results. New research suggests that exfoliated cells may be investigated further for epigenetic changes and other genetic mutations, as well as screening populations with exfoliative cytology-assisted cytomorphology [10].

10.1.5. Brush biopsy

To improve exfoliative cytology, the technique of brush biopsy may be used. Inadequate or inaccurate, negative or no abnormality, atypical or abnormal and positive or cell atypia/carcinoma are the main results that may be achieved from a sample. Brush biopsy success depends on its correct usage, whereby a sample must penetrate the whole epithelium until basement membrane, effectively leading to 'pinpoint bleeding' on sample taking. Shallow samples are therefore inaccurate and may yield false negative results. Although Brush biopsies have had promising positive predictive values/positive likelihood ratios in predicting dysplasia and/or cancer cells in dysplastic and/or SCC lesions, their false negative results have also been presented in several cases and so wisely, conventional methods (scalpel/punch biopsy) should never be superseded by brush biopsy technique [61]. Recently, advances in brush biopsy include using the assistance of matrix-assisted laser absorption/ionisation time to detect changes between malignant and non-malignant cells by analysing their complete mass spectra [4] to diagnose early cancer cell changes.

10.1.6. Scalpel and punch biopsy

Although both are surgical techniques, the conventional scalpel biopsy removes all layers of the epithelium and enters connective tissue and can be used to extend the biopsy sample where required. The punch biopsy is a more cleaner form of sampling and should be limited to small lesions, more anterior based or extraoral. Scalpel biopsies may be incisional or excisional and importantly should be carried out before treatment is given and ideally be carried out by the same team, also delivering treatment (healing of biopsy may obscure primary lesion location). It should contain the most suspicious area, be large and deep enough for comfortable histopathological diagnosis, be a representative sample of the disease in progress (multiple biopsies may be required here), is of excellent quality (not crushed) and fixed in formal saline to prevent autolysis. Importantly, where results come back negative and the line of doubt for malignancy still exists, biopsies should be challenged and repeated. Other factors include the informed consent of the patient, the reliability of patient-clinician interrelationship and the management of post-operative complications of biopsy where they occur. A biopsy serves to confirm or change the cancer diagnosis with histopathological clarity and grade stage of disease, indicate cancer type and describe if there is local invasion to bone, nerve and muscle. Incisional biopsies may predispose to seeding particularly in areas such as the salivary glands. Some reports have even highlighted that metastasis to lymph nodes by SCC was predisposed by biopsy, whereby cancer cells have potential to reach peripheral blood after the procedure. However, the importance of this investigation remains vital.

http://dx.doi.org/10.5772/intechopen.71887

10.1.7. Fine needle aspiration biopsy (FNA)

Lymph nodes and other superficial areas or lesions may be assessed using FNA, a method using a fine-bore needle to aspirate cells and other materials such as blood, cyst fluid and pus for cytological examination. Ultrasound or CT-guided FNA may be more advantageous in giving accuracy to the location of the sample. When assessing metastasis to a lymph node, other features include size of deposits, anatomical level of involvement, extracapsular spread and presence of embolization/permeation of perinodal lymphatics [62].

10.1.8. Sentinel lymph node biopsy

Sentinel lymph node biopsy assesses the first lymph node that the primary tumour most likely can drain/spread to and is important in correctly staging Oral Cancer. Techniques for this procedure include applying a radioactive tracer material and using conventional radiography to locate the lymph node in question. Blue dye may be used during surgery and the lymph node is then removed and assessed. Elective neck dissection, however, remains a more strengthened path to treatment as evidence suggests that even with negative sentinel lymph node results, metastasis could occur on nonsentinel lymph nodes and through bilateral drainage in the head and neck, thus predisposing to metastatic development.

10.1.9. Examination under general anaesthesia

Patients may require more thorough investigation of the mouth, upper aero-digestive tract and areas of the nose pharynx, larynx and oesophagus in obscured, small or untraceable lesions. Lesions that cannot be seen visually or palpated may require this procedure. These also include lesions with an enlarged lymph node where no visible primary neoplasm or margins are ill-defined. Random biopsies may be helpful in areas of nasopharynx, base of tongue and hypopharynx as well as tonsil, fossa of Rosenmuller and ipsilateral tonsillectomy.

10.1.10. Imaging

Conventional radiography—orthopantomogram, and intra-oral radiographs maybe useful in the initial detection of SCC or other tumours in the oral cavity. Chest X-ray is an important primary investigation to assess pulmonary or airway disease in the lungs, hilar lymph nodes, ribs and vertebrae, as well as the detection of any infectious or metastatic disease of the lungs. Ultrasound can be used in assessing lymph nodes, guiding FNA and helps in diagnosing swellings. Doppler-blood flow studies are important in planning radial free forearm flaps. Nasoendoscopy, Laryngoscopy and Panendoscopy investigations are utilised to visualise upper air passages and the pharynx as well as the latter being used under GA to examine trachea, bronchi and oesophagus. Computerised tomography (CT) and Cone beam computerised tomography (CBCT) are vital in the diagnosis of Oral Cancer and help to delineate the origin, extension and size of lesion as well as degree of bone invasion by tumour and in analysing extent of jaw lesions determining lymph node involvement cervically or distant metastasis. CBCT is advantageous with reduced radiation doses, rapid scan times and unique oral and maxillofacial display systems. Where there is metastasis in the oral cavity, imaging serves to find the occult primary tumour. Dual energy CT improves tumour margin visibility by providing an image that has a high tissue contrast and image noise reduction (particularly useful for reducing dental filling artefact close to tumour study and improving reconstruction) [63]. Standard magnetic resonance imaging (MRI) is beneficial in soft tissue analysis of neurovascular bundles, and cervical lymph node involvement. MRI serves to delineate specific differences between tissues of neoplasms and inflammation as well as normal tissue. Advanced MRI techniques may also be necessary and include spectroscopy, perfusion imaging and diffusion weighted imaging where the latter can be used to detect tumours, assess their character and analyse metastatic lymph node staging [64]. Additional gadolinium-based intravenous contrast can also aid in assessing tumour extension.

10.1.11. Nuclear medicine

Positron emission tomography (PET) scan is utilised to provide 3d imaging in the investigation for accurate tumour localisation, discovery of metastatic disease and occult lymph node involvement where a radioactive drug is injected such as 18-fluorodeoxyglucose that is taken up by cells with increased metabolic activity (cancer cells). PET fusion scans are also beneficial in the evaluation of a patient with metastatic lymph nodes particularly where the primary tumour cannot be found. The use of PET/CT combination serves to stage head and neck malignancies, lymphadenopathies and to exclude malignancy in lesions that are not fully determined by CT [57]. Bone scans show any abnormal areas of bone, where a radioactive substance is injected into a vein and hot spots are revealed such as Technetium 99 bone scans that are useful in determining bone metabolic activity and active growth or infection.

10.1.12. Saliva

The role of saliva analysis in diagnosing Oral Cancer is a new field, and a unique one due to the contact relationship between Oral Cancer and saliva composition. Indeed, many changes have been found in saliva composition among Oral Cancer patients compared to healthy controls. Such compositional changes include increase in total sugar, free and protein-bound sialic acid, sodium, calcium and calcium-binding protein, albumin and lactate dehydrogenase. Immunological alterations within saliva have also been detected and include presence of Immunoglobulin C and increased insulin-like growth factor, matrix metalloproteinases and Interleukin 8 and 1B. Epithelial tumours markers such as CYFRA 21-1 and genetic alterations such as presence of HA3 oncogene, Micro RNAs 125a and 200a, and DUSP1, a regulator of cell proliferation, have all been noted within saliva of Oral Cancer patients compared to controls thus allowing saliva to become a future examination in the detection of Oral Cancer.

10.1.13.Blood

Blood samples may become new aids in the diagnosis of Oral Cancer. Mineral levels of iron and selenium (low in Oral Cancer patients) and copper (high in Oral Cancer patients) may be useful adjuncts. Serological parameters include squamous cell carcinoma-associated antigen, carcinoembryonic antigen, inhibitor of apoptosis fragments and cytokeratin fragments as well as Annexin A1 [19]. Recently, it has bene proposed that the combination of Serum Il-6 mRNA and Salivary Il-8 mRNA has almost complete sensitivity and specificity in the detection of Oral Cancer [10].

10.1.14. Micro RNAs

MiR-21, MiR-125b and MiR-203, for example, have all been highlighted as potentially new diagnostic aids not only in diagnosing SCC but also in the differentiation of tumour subtypes. Tumours from different locations in the oral cavity (base of tongue and tonsil) were shown to express different Micro RNAs thus, where tumour location is unknown or primary origin of nodal metastasis is unclear, the study of Mi-RNAs may becoming a promising field. MiR-21 and MiR-375, in particular, have been detected in cytological samples in people with early tongue SCC compared to controls and thus may have a role in the accurate detection of this disease while MiR-139-5p was found to be reduced in saliva patients of tongue SCC compared to controls. MiR-184 in plasma was elevated in patients with tongue SCC compared to controls and returned to normal upon removal of tumour [21].

10.1.15. Others

The analysis of cellular proliferation and DNA ploidy with flow cytometry may be a promising new field as detection of aneuploid DNA content within cancer cells is an important biological characteristic. The use of 5-bromodeoxyuridine to detect cellular proliferation particularly in poorly differentiated SCC may be a new method of investigation as well as differentiating tumours with increased lymph node involvement [65]. Biomarkers are also a new and important field in the detection of Oral Cancer. Along with TNM staging, the depiction of Oral Cancer using specific and unique features to determine prognosis are all important non-negligible addition to Oral Cancer diagnosis.

11. Clinical features of SCC

SCC often appears as a raised, firm swelling with rolled margins and a granular floor, or as a plaque-like lesion with irregular, roughened or verrucous areas of mucosal thickening. As they continue to enlarge, they may become ulcerated and protruded masses that have irregular and indurated borders with necrosis centrally. Pain may arise as lesion gets more infiltrative and nerves become involved. SCC development often includes the lower lip due to sunlight exposure and the lateral margins of the tongue and the floor of the mouth (non-keratinised areas) are often preceded by an Erythroplakic lesion. Other areas include the posterolateral margin of the tongue which is often termed the 'coffin corner', usually detected as late-stage disease with metastatic involvement and the alveolus and gingivae are often affected in the mandibular premolar and molar regions. The buccal mucosa unfortunately presents with one of the most aggressive clinical courses of SCC and occurs in the areas of the buccal commissures and retromolar areas. Finally, carcinomas in the palate may affect both the soft and hard region and may be of minor salivary gland origin or extending from the maxillary antrum [56].

Spread of SCC depends on location and is related to anatomical features of that area. Cancers of the lip, for example, invade adjacent skin, orbicular muscle and when increased in size, the buccal mucosa, mandible and mental nerve. Those tumours of the tongue usually arise on lateral and posterior surfaces and eventually invade the floor of the mouth, root of tongue and causes fixation. Floor of the mouth SCC further extends into the sublingual gland, mid-line muscle and extends towards the gingivae and mandible. Tumours of the buccal mucosa rapidly invade underlying muscles and may even penetrate skin. Other areas include the hard palate where the maxillary antrum may become involved. The retromolar region often involves the adjacent buccal mucosa, anterior tonsillar pillars, maxilla, pterygomandibular space, medial pterygoid muscle and buccinator. The mandible often is affected in the body and then spreads to the ramus.

12. Associated signs and symptoms of Oral Cancer development

These include but are not limited to the development of premalignant lesions, non-healing oral ulceration, non-healing extraction sockets, swellings of the mouth and neck, firm and fixed lesions, loosening of one or more teeth, altered dental occlusion, jaw pain, ear pain (ear pain in relation to SCC of the tongue in particular), neck stiffness, regional or cervical lymph-adenopathy (30–80% of patients may present with lymph node enlargement as initial presentation), difficulty in mastication, swallowing and speech, paraesthesia, voice hoarseness and temporomandibular joint (TMJ) disorder symptoms. Indeed, pain is an important factor that is associated with the Oral Cancer directly and in metastatic lesions to the oral cavity that can affect nerves. Nasopharyngeal tumours often present with TMJ disorder-like symptoms such as trismus, deviation of the jaw and headaches. Paraneoplastic phenomena may be also be evident in cases of SCC and include the presentation of hypercalcemia and melanosis. Oral paraneoplastic melanosis is a newly described entity that may present with SCC, direct or adjacent to tumour where there is melanin pigmentation that is not histologically associated with tumour histology, rather a distinct entity of unknown aetiology with its presence being a possible diagnostic aid in SCC [66].

13. Histological variants of SCC

SCC can vary widely in histological pattern and other microscopic features. Some SCCs are infiltrated with eosinophils, and melanocytes and some may resemble other tumours such as large cell malignant lymphoma. Immunohistochemistry also varies for SCCs where most are invariably positive for keratin. CK 5, 6, 8, 13, 18 and 19 are all varyingly expressed within lesions where CK13, for example, is associated with metastasis. Desmosome-related proteins and involucrin expression (a marker of terminal differentiation of squamous epithelial cells and keratinisation) are also important immunohistochemical findings (**Figure 1**).

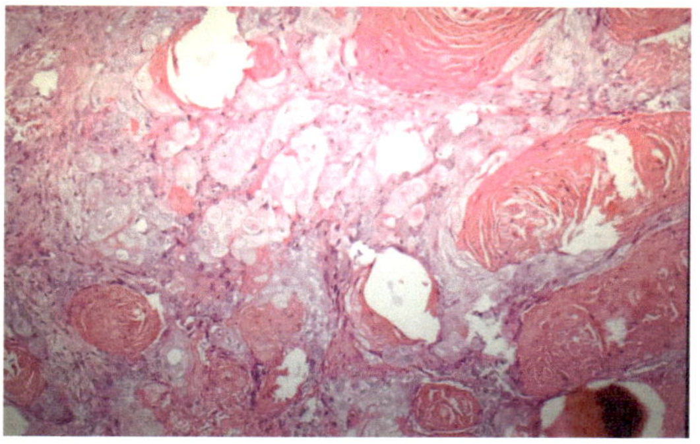

Figure 1. Keratin pearls and nests of well-differentiated invasive (keratinising) squamous cell carcinoma (40×).

13.1. Verrucous SCC or Ackerman's tumour

Verrucous SCC or Ackerman's tumour does not usually metastasise (although can invade bone and nerves) and is often seen on the alveolar ridge, mandibular sulci or buccal mucosa in patients who use smokeless tobacco. Clinically, it resembles an exophytic lesions with papillary growth that can become infected. Histologically, there are bulbous rete ridges that are swollen and increased in volume with smooth rounded outlines, blunt invasion from a wide advancing front and minimal cytological atypia (**Figure 2**).

13.2. Papillary SCC

Papillary SCC is another variant that shows paraorthokeratosis or orthokeratosis, significant cellular atypia and micro abscesses at the tips of bulbous rete ridges. The tumour may resemble verrucous carcinoma in its blunt invasion or may be single celled or island cell invasion however often contains HPV infection and is more present in the oropharynx in elderly patients.

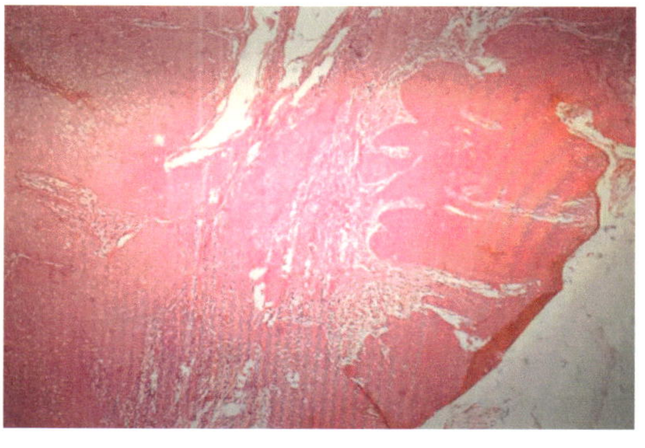

Figure 2. Verrucous squamous cell carcinoma showing pushing borders (4×).

13.3. Adenoid squamous cell carcinoma, acantholytic or pseudoglandular SCC

Adenoid squamous cell carcinoma, acantholytic or pseudoglandular SCC commonly arises on the lower lip (probably due to UV radiation) with an aggressive pattern compared to its skin counterpart. There is proliferation of malignant squamous cells and acantholysis with pseudoglandular structures. This SCC may be misdiagnosed as an adenocarcinoma, adenosquamous cell carcinoma or mucoepidermoid carcinoma.

13.4. Adenosquamous cell carcinoma

Adenosquamous cell carcinoma is mainly found in the posterior tongue with poor prognosis (65% risk of metastasis). This variant is a proliferation of squamous cells with formation of duct-like structures containing mucous cells and basaloid epithelial cells.

13.5. Basaloid SCC

Basaloid SCC is an aggressive variant with presence of solid tumour islands, peripheral palisading, thick basement membrane as well as basal lamina material. Cystic spaces are often present and such may resemble adenoid cystic carcinoma or ameloblastoma.

13.6. Squamous proliferation with neoplastic goblet cells

Squamous proliferation with neoplastic goblet cells should also not be confused with clear cell carcinoma [4]. Small cell carcinoma may be pure or has a squamous component with aggressive nature (similar to lung presentation). NUT midline carcinoma is a newly recognised type of carcinoma with molecular changes to NUT gene on chromosome 15 affecting midline structures of the head and neck. Histologically, there are islands of undifferentiated carcinoma with keratinisation with positivity for CK8/18 and CK5/6 respectively.

13.7. Clear cell SCC

Clear cell SCC is a rare histological entity where epithelial malignant cells exhibit this appearance due to degeneration and accumulation of intracellular fluid and contain glycogen. Histologically, these tumours are Periodic acid Schiff (PAS), mucicarmine and S100 negative, CK8 and CK18 positive with squamous differentiation with absence of vasculature or haemorrhaging (**Figure 3**).

13.8. Lymphoepithelioma-like carcinoma

Lymphoepithelioma-like carcinoma is a poorly differentiated or undifferentiated SCC with prominent reactive lymphoplasmacytic infiltrate resembling its non-keratinising nasopharyngeral counterpart and rarely can affect the oral tissues such as the tongue. Malignant cells contain vascular nuclei, prominent nucleoli, pale chromatin and ill-defined cell borders. Pseudovascular SCC may be misdiagnosed as angiosarcoma or giant-cell carcinoma and immunohistochemistry for cytokeratins or endothelial markers should differentiate these.

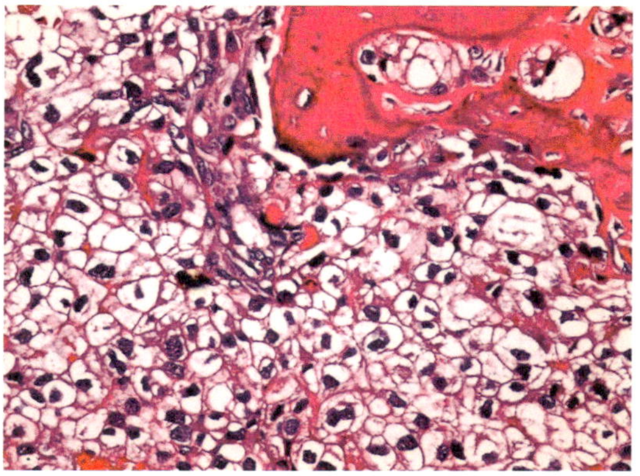

Figure 3. Clear cell SCC. Sheets of cells with dark nuclei, small nucleoli and abundant clear cytoplasm. There are scattered mitoses. The tumour is infiltrating bone at the top right of the figure (40×). Courtesy of Prof. Elhassan and Prof. Elimairi.

14. Metastasis, recurrence and survival

SCC of the oral cavity invades locally before metastasising to regional lymph nodes and distant sites. Features that aid metastasis of SCC include its location (high risk posterior tongue, oropharynx, floor of mouth), microscopic differentiation (poorly differentiated), depth of invasion or tumour thickness (more than 9 mm) and presence of inflammatory component. SCC often proliferates as single cells locally or as islands and cords. Those tumours with bulbous rete ridges often invade slowly with less metastasis. Once there is lymphovascular, perineural or bone invasion, local and distant metastasis may be present with recurrence high and possibly poor survival. The submental and submandibular lymph nodes are often the first to be affected and tumours of the posterior tongue often drain to the jugulodigastric or tonsillar lymph nodes and may be bilateral. Distant metastasis includes the mediastinal lymph nodes, lungs, breast and kidneys with bone and liver being affected less commonly. Cervical lymph node metastasis by oral SCC can sometimes exhibit peculiar histological changes such as cystic degeneration that can thus resemble branchial cyst with malignant changes and foreign body giant cell reaction around keratin without presence of tumour cells.

15. Metastasis of distant cancers to the oral cavity

Metastasis from infrabodily regions to the oral cavity affects the hard and soft tissues and carries with it its own sequelae and important signs and symptoms. Metastatic cancer cells, most often carcinomas but may also be sarcomas, enter the circulatory system by a process of intravasation and leave by extravasation, adhere to vessels and arrest due to their large size. Colonisation of tissues then quickly occurs by metastatic cells as well as their adaptability to the local environment with buildup of neovascularity. The bone, i.e., jaw and in particular the mandible, is the most common location affected by metastatic cancer in the head and neck due to chemoattraction and release of cytokines released by it that attracts metastatic cell growth but soft tissues are affected as well. Indeed, osteolytic lesions such as breast and myeloma and osteoblastic lesions such as prostate, commonly can present in the mandible or maxillary regions. Other metastatic possibilities include the kidney, thyroid, lung, cervix, bladder, liver, colon and stomach. Batsons vertebral venous plexus may be a route for cancers to reach the jaws without affecting the lungs. Metastasis to the soft tissues is mainly to the attached gingivae and the tongue and often resembles a benign exophytic or polypoid lesion with high vascularity.

Signs and symptoms of metastatic to the jaws include pain, increasing tooth mobility, swellings, paraesthesia (numb chin syndrome) and other features such as delayed healing of extraction socket, progressive trismus and other symptoms that mimic TMJ dysfunction. Radiographic features include lytic radiolucent lesions, moth-eaten appearance of bone, resorption of teeth and mimicry of periodontal disease. These, however, are often late presenting signs of metastasis and earlier disease may require other investigations such as bone scintigraphy. Soft tissues signs and symptoms include swellings with haemorrhagic tendency, ulceration and necrosis. Finally, the salivary glands should also be noted where metastatic cancers of the salivary glands represent about 8% of all tumours to the gland, the parotid being the main one affected. Commonly, metastasis to the glands is from the head and neck region itself mainly SCC and melanoma. Other tumours include renal, lungs, breast and prostate cancer. Signs and symptoms include swellings, paraesthesia and facial weakness. For a metastatic tumour to be diagnosed, criteria must be reached that includes finding a primary tumour that is histologically accurate to the metastatic sample and that the neoplasm does not involve histopathological appearance of oral tumours [7].

16. Other types of Oral Cancer

16.1. Odontogenic malignancies

Odontogenic tumours are often benign and local, however although rare, odontogenic malignancies can also occur and are discussed in this paragraph. Peripheral intraosseous SCCs (solid or cystic form) are thought to arise from either odontogenic epithelium or incisive canal epithelium and thus initiate in the jaws with exclusion of secondary spread or metastasis to site. Other intraosseous odontogenic carcinomas include mucoepidermoid carcinoma presenting at the angle of the mandible with histological display of squamous differentiation, mucous cells and mucicarmine positivity.

Ameloblastomas, a common and usually benign odontogenic tumour, can however metastasise, tracking to the lungs (through spill into lymphatic/blood vessels or possibly suggested aspiration of tumour fragments during surgery) leading to multifocal deposits. Through dedifferentiation of cells, ameloblastic carcinomas may also develop either out of an ameloblastoma or occur as de novo displaying an aggressive neoplasm overgrowing the ameloblastic component with great cytological atypia, mitotic activity with basilar hyperplasia as well as perineural invasion. Low grade spindle ameloblastic carcinoma is another form displaying cellular stroma and fibroblastic cells. Ghost cell odontogenic carcinomas are often locally invasive but can metastasise to the orbit, cranium or lungs, and are a form of ameloblastic carcinomatous differentiation with histological positivity for enamel matrix protein amelogenin and display of ameloblastic columnar cell pattern at periphery. Other findings include sheets of basaloid cells and stratified squamous epithelium with ghost cell keratinisation (enlarged epithelial cell with eosinophilic cytoplasm). Clear cell odontogenic carcinoma may also show peripheral palisaded ameloblastic columnar cells and show budded cords, islands of malignant epithelial cells as well as clear cells (cells with abundant pale cytoplasm with distinct cell borders). Clear cell odontogenic carcinoma should be differentially diagnosed from calcifying epithelial odontogenic tumour, metastatic renal carcinoma, clear cell variant of mucoepidermoid carcinoma and clear cell squamous cell carcinoma. Ameloblastic fibrocarcoma usually occurs de novo but can arise from ameloblastic fibroma, presenting in young age groups in the mandible with extraosseous soft tissue extension and present radiologically as an expansile radiolucency. Histologically, there is benign odontogenic epithelium with malignant connective tissue cells. Even more so, dentine and or enamel differentiation may also occur leading to the term ameloblastic dentinosarcoma and/or ameloblastic odontosarcoma. The keratocyst and dentigerous cyst are the commonest odontogenic cysts that can develop malignancy where the former often is present in older age groups as an asymptomatic or otherwise painful pericoronal lesion associated with an unerupted mandibular wisdom tooth as well as canines and the latter may arise within lesion or after surgeries [67].

16.2. Osteosarcomas

Osteosarcomas are primary bone tumours of mesenchymal origin and are rare in the head and neck region however when do present, are often in the jaws around the 4th decade of life (compared to infrabody osteosarcoma which occurs around the 2nd decade and associated growth spurts), and are aggressive lesions (although jaw osteosarcoma has better prognosis compared to other locations due to less haematogenous spread and better histological differentiation). Possible aetiopathological factors exist such as genetical pleomorphisms (inactivation of the retinoblastoma gene), bone dysplasias and previous radiation therapy. Radiographically, bone undergoes a typical sunray appearance and widening of periodontal ligament space (Grittmans sign). Histologically, malignant spindle cells are found producing osteoid and immature bone with possible cartilaginous differentiation (**Figure 4**).

16.3. Lymphomas (B, T and NK cell)

Where cases of non-Hodgkin's Lymphoma (NHL) do occur in the oral cavity, 70% of them present in Waldeyer's ring (tonsil, adenoid, tongue base, nasopharynx) lack in ulceration and are present with dysphagia, airway obstruction, Eustachian tube blockage and neck

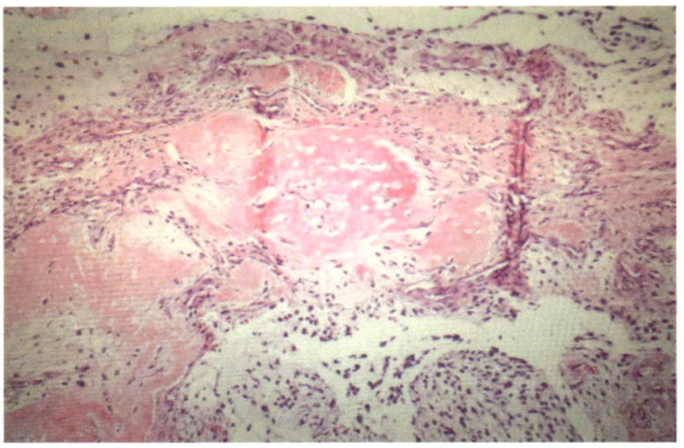

Figure 4. Osteosarcoma: sheets of malignant cells with adjoining osteoid and new bone (4×).

involvement. Those that do occur in the oral soft tissues are usually to the buccal vestibule, gingivae and hard palate as well as centrally within the jaws, presenting as a rapidly growing tumour with ulceration and necrosis sometimes accompanied with an erythematous purplish appearance. The different types of NHL that can affect the oral cavity are summarised below.

16.3.1. Diffuse large B-cell lymphoma (DLBCL)

DLBCL often presents in elder age groups (6th and 7th decade) as a painless mass. Histologically, centroblastic, anaplastic, and immunoblastic and T cell/histiocyte rich subtypes exist. Plasmablastic B cell lymphoma is a DLBCL variant most commonly in HIV affected persons and usually affects the buccal-gingival mucosa. Histologically they are CD20− and CD138+ lack of cancerous plasma cells but existence of plasmablastic morphology.

16.3.2. Burkett's lymphoma

This is an aggressive, highly proliferative tumour (nearly 100% Ki-67 proliferation fraction) occurring as either endemic (Africa, 1st, 2nd decade in life, 95% EBV + associated), sporadic (no geographical or age predilection, <30% EBV + associated) or HIV-related cases (25–40% EBV + associated) and almost uniquely presenting in the jaws. Classical histology includes a starry sky appearance (scattered macrophages) with round medium-sized blastic lymphoid cells that contain coarse chromatin and multiple nucleoli with CD10, 19, 20, and 22 positivity. Genetically, Burkett's lymphoma is known to be associated with c-myc translocation and 100% Bcl-6 hypermutation, as well as being BCL2 (anti-apoptotic) negative.

16.3.3. Mantle cell lymphoma

Rare cases have been reported in particular palatally masked by prosthetic appliances in elderly patients. Histologically, these lymphomas contain small lymphoid cells with hyperchromatism and CD-19, 20 and cyclin D1 positivity. These tumours are also CD5, CD10 and CD23 negative and BCL-2 positive.

16.3.4. Follicular lymphoma

Often in salivary glands, malignant lymphocytes are in follicular patterns with progressive destruction of salivary gland structure. Follicular lymphoma is also highly positive for the anti-apoptotic protein BCL-2 positive as well as CD-20.

16.3.5. Mucosal associated lymphoid tissue (MALT) lymphoma

Another associated salivary gland lymphoma is MALT lymphoma usually associated with Sjogrens syndrome patients and thus has a female predominance. This tumour contains T cells, B cells as well as plasma cells and macrophages often with a slow course.

16.3.6. Mycosis fungoides

Also known as cutaneous T cell lymphoma, only a handful of oral cases have been reported in the literature and often occur after skin lesions. The tongue is a favourable site where ulceration, indurated leukoplakic-like lesions and erosions occur. Malignant proliferation of helper (CD-4) T lymphocytes and suppressor T lymphocytes occurs with histological dense infiltrate of pleomorphic lymphocytes and Pautrier's microabscesses.

16.3.7. Peripheral T cell lymphoma

While these may simulate NK/T cell lymphoma, they are a rare type of T cell lymphoma and even rarer to occur in the oral cavity. These often occur at elder age and immunohistochemistry distinguishes them by their CD56 and CD20 negativity and CD3 positivity (**Figures 5** and **6**).

16.3.8. Lethal midline granuloma/natural killer T cell lymphoma

As its name, this tumour often has an extremely rapid course with terrible prognosis. Typically originating in the nasal cavity, perforation intraorally to the palate as well as extension to

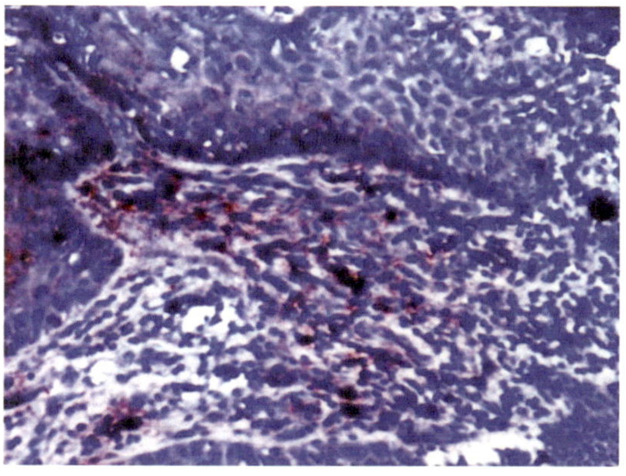

Figure 5. Peripheral T cell lymphoma. Immunohistochemistry: cells negative for CD56.

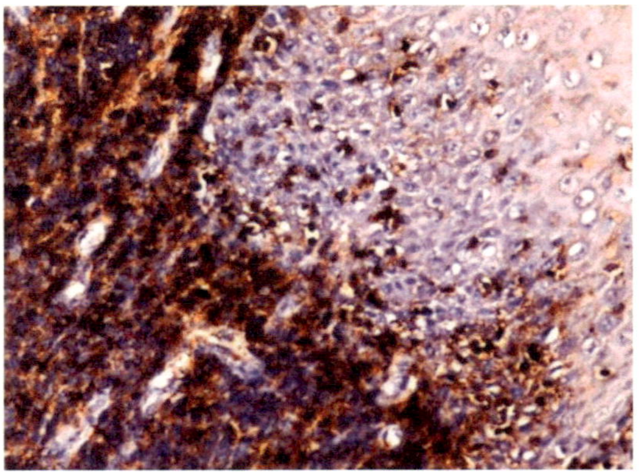

Figure 6. Peripheral T cell lymphoma. Cells positive for CD3. Courtesy of Prof. Elhassan and Prof. Elimairi.

midface region occurs often in young males with an unclear aetiology. Initially, non-specific rhinitis and/or sinusitis as well as epistaxis confuses the initial clinical picture; however, progressive facial swelling and deep necrotic ulceration in the midline of the face ensues, leading to oronasal destruction and systemic manifestations. Histologically, there are bizarre lymphocytes with large and hyperchromatic nuclei.

16.4. Plasmacytomas (intramedullary, extramedullary or multiple myeloma)

In the oral cavity, malignant plasma cells can rarely give rise to solitary proliferations that are present either in the bone (intramedullary), in soft tissues (extramedullary) or as part of multifocal disseminated disease known as multiple myeloma [68]. The latter is characterised by other systemic features such as M proteins, bone lytic lesions, kidney failure, hepato and splenomegaly with progressive hypercalcaemia and hyperviscosity, as well aplastic anaemia with concurrent infections. Oral lesions can develop in up to 30% of patients with multiple myeloma and can be present as jaw pain, pathological fractures, swelling, paraesthaesia and tooth complications such as mobility and resorption. Radiologically, bone loss and osteolytic lesions in the jaws may be evident giving a punched out appearance. Painless soft tissue ulceration and swelling may be evident. A not uncommon feature is amyloidosis relating to the disease and can present as macroglossia, papules, nodules and plaque-like lesions in the soft tissues as well as rarely in the salivary glands [69]. Histologically, clusters, nodules or sheets of malignant plasma cells in an interstitial, focal or diffuse manner in a hypercellular marrow are evident with osteclastic activity and CD138 positivity. Plasma cells with Russell bodies (intracytoplasmic hyaline inclusions) may also be seen and are termed Mott cells as well as other histological features including Dutcher bodies.

16.5. Kaposi's sarcoma

Kaposi's sarcoma, a low grade tumour of endothelial vascular cell arises as either classic or sporadic (Mediterranean and Eastern Europe), endemic (Africa), epidemic (HIV associated) or immunosuppression forms (transplant, immunosuppressive therapy such as Rituximab or Corticosteroid) [70]. Kaposi's sarcoma develops in the skin, lymphatics, mucous membranes and viscera such as the lungs, stomach and liver. A combination of aetiopathological factors exists, most importantly of which is HHV-8 seroconversion that is thought to lead to the Warburg effect among cells, promotes release of pro-inflammatory cytokines and allows immune breakdown. Immunosuppression plays a strong role in development of Kaposi's sarcoma as well as chronic inflammation. Up to 70% of HIV patients can develop Kaposi's sarcoma in the oral cavity and 20% of any associated pattern of Kaposi's sarcoma will manifest in the mouth.

Orally, Kaposi's sarcoma lesions, which are commonly due to the epidemic and immunosuppression forms, are often round, single or multiple swellings that are flat, papuled or nodular, most likely to appear on the palate and gingivae (sometimes mimicking gingival hyperplasia), but rarely can present in the lips, tongue and buccal mucosa. It is often purple, red, brown or blue colour and may be associated with secondary bleeding, ulceration and necrosis if long standing. Bone involvement and tooth mobility may also arise. Histologically, Kaposi's sarcoma lesions contain spindle-shaped malignant cells, abnormal vessels (stellate or ecstatic patterns), vascular slit-like spaces, extravasated erythrocytes, haemosiderin laden macrophages, hyaline globules and chronic inflammatory infiltrate with plasma cells and lymphocytes. Anaplastic, pyogenic granuloma-like and lymphangioma-like histological variants exist. Endothelial cell markers CD31 and CD34 are positive as well as presence of vascular endothelial growth factor 3 relates to lymphatic differentiation within Kaposi's sarcoma. MMPs and IL6 presence are associated with angiogenesis; however, no chromosomal abnormalities are known [71].

16.6. Ewing's sarcoma

Unfortunately, not an uncommon aggressive tumour present in childhood or adolescence (more commonly among Caucasians), Ewing's sarcoma carries a poor prognosis with likely metastasis upon clinical presentation. Most likely derived from neuroectodermal cells, Ewing's sarcoma may also have a reticular and mesenchymal cell origin. Genetically, the translocation t (11.22) (q24:12) is present in over 90% of cases leading to fusion of the Ewing's sarcoma/Friend leukaemia integration 1 transcription factor that gives rise to a strong oncogene. Other genetic alterations include P16 activation and p53 suppression. Histologically, Ewing's sarcoma consists of small round cell tumours that are CD99 positive and neural marker negative and exhibits intracellular glycogen granules and abundant intermediate filaments. Head and Neck Ewing's sarcoma accounts for 3% of cases but 10% of all bone malignancies of mandible. Patients present with a hard or elastic soft bone swelling are most likely in posterior mandible but can occur in maxilla and maxillary sinus, gingival swelling, pain or toothache, dental abscess, paraesthesia as well as dental disturbances that include destruction of dental follicles, premature exfoliation, tooth mobility and resorption. Overlying mucosal may appear normal but can show erythema or ulceration. Radiographically, the tumour is radiotransparent with irregular margins and no sclerotic reaction [72].

16.7. Malignant melanoma

Arising from primary malignant transformation of melanocytes in the basal layer (and less commonly from immature melanocytes in lamina propria), malignant melanoma represents a rare entity (0.5% of Oral Cancer) in the oral cavity with very poor prognosis. Melanoma may arise in a background of benign oral pigmentation such as nevus but can occur de novo with absence of any existing pigmented lesion and often presents in the hard palate, gingivae, buccal mucosa or retromolar region as either a macule, papule or exophytic lesion. Rarely, it may secondarily metastasise from skin melanoma to the oral cavity. Tumours are often painless, irregular and represent mottled pigmentation that is of a brown to black nature with lesional bleeding. Invasion to deeper structures, satellite tumours and metastasis to local and distant lymph nodes occurs rapidly. The aggressiveness of this tumour is both in relation to its melanotic progenitor cells, when replicate provides new melanotic amplified cells with an extremely high proliferative rate, but also to its histopathological growth pattern which allows malignant cells to invade along the whole of the basal cell layer of epithelium, followed by vertical growth of malignant cells into the lamina propria thus spreading widely undisturbed before being clinically visible. Genetically, melanocortin receptor 1 polymorphisms (associated with less DNA repair and apoptosis of damaged melanocytes), CKit proto-oncogene overexpression and altered cadherin cell adhesion molecules (increased N cadherin expression promotes cell proliferation, migration and invasive potential) are implicated in the development of this tumour. Interestingly, a cancer promoting cycle occurs during melanin biosynthesis whereby melanin degradation leads to the release of reactive oxygen species, formation of quinines and other products that are mutagenic and produce melanocyte instability. Histologically, melanoma cells are highly mitotic with eosinphilic nuclei in either solid or loose arrangement with variable melanin expression. Melanin expression can also be detected within macrophages and extracellularly, sometimes so much as to hide cancer cell morphology. Absence of pigment in melanoma cells reveals another variant that is amelanotic melanoma with an even poorer prognosis than its counterpart, owing to its delayed diagnosis [73].

16.8. Collision, bimorphic and hybrid tumours

Two or more primary tumours may rarely grow alongside one another with no or limited histological intersection, termed; collision tumours. Often these consist of carcinomas and sarcomas, sarcomas and lymphomas or two types of carcinomas. Cases in the literature including SCC growth include alongside ameloblastomas, pleomorphic adenomas, salivary duct carcinomas, thyroid carcinomas and melanomas have been reported. A bimorphic tumour consists of two types of tissues or cells, one of malignant cell origin and one form often considered non-cancer proliferation such as the stromal background (thought to be a reaction to presence of epithelial carcinoma cells) seen within spindle cell SCC or pseudosarcoma. However, the latter tumour also delivers other histological concepts, such as tumour cell polyclonal originality, where both epithelial and spindle cells are originated from different stem cell lines and monoclonal originality whereby mutagenic changes at some point lead to spindle cell formation within the tumour or just dedifferentiation of original tumour cells. Neuroectodermal tumour of infancy is another example of a biphasic tumour consisting of both neuroblastic cells and large melanin containing epithelial cells. Hybrid tumours consists of two or more tumour tissue in a single neoplasm and arises within the same topography of lesion such as sarcomatous change within a carcinoma (carcinosarcoma) [74]. It may be of note that infections and synchronous SCC growth have also been reported such as tuberculosis and SCC growth within one anatomical space and Paracoccidioidiomycosis alongside an oesophageal carcinoma.

Author details

Imad Elimairi*, Amel Sami and Badreldin Yousef

*Address all correspondence to: imad56@gmail.com

National Ribat University, Khartoum, Sudan

References

[1] Niu LX et al. Prognostic factors of squamous cell carcinoma of the buccal mucosa: A retrospective study of 168 cases in Journal of Oral Maxillofacial Surgery. American Association of Oral and Maxillofacial Surgeons. 2014;**72**(11):2344-2350. DOI: 10.1016/j.joms.2014.05.021

[2] Scully C, Bedi R. Ethnicity and oral cancer. Lancet Oncology. 2000 Sep;**1**(1):37-42

[3] Tabatabaeifar S et al. Investigating a case of possible field cancerization in oral squamous cell carcinoma by the use of next-generation sequencing. Oral Oncology. 2017;**68**:74-80. DOI: 10.1016/j.oraloncology.2017.03.018

[4] Weinstock YE, Iii IA, Dierks EJ. Pitfalls in determining head and neck surgical margins. Oral and Maxillofacial Surgery Clinics of NA. 2014;**26**(2):151-162. DOI: 10.1016/j.coms.2014.01.003

[5] Subramaniam N, Balasubramanian D. Adverse pathologic features in early oral squamous cell carcinoma and the role of postoperative radiotherapy d a review. Oral Surgery, Oral Medicine, Oral Pathology, and Oral Radiology. 2017;**124**(1):24-31. DOI: 10.1016/j.oooo.2017.03.002

[6] Wagner VP, Webber P, Curra M. 'Bryne' s grading system predicts poor disease-specific survival of oral squamous cell carcinoma: A comparative study among different histologic grading systems. Oral Surgery, Oral Medicine, Oral Pathology, and Oral Radiology. 2017;**123**(6):688-696. DOI: 10.1016/j.oooo.2017.02.012

[7] Vega LG, Dipasquale J. Head and neck manifestations of distant carcinomas. Oral and Maxillofacial Surgery Clinics of NA. 2008;**20**(4):609-623. DOI: 10.1016/j.coms.2008.06.003

[8] Kaneko T, Dehari H, Sasaki T. Hypoxia induced epithelial-mesenchymal transition is regulated by phosphorylation of GSK3-b via PI3 K/Akt signalling in oral squamous cell carcinoma. Oral Surgery, Oral Medicine, Oral Pathology, and Oral Radiology. 2016;**122**(6):719-730. DOI: 10.1016/j.oooo.2016.06.008

[9] Van Der Waal I. Potentially malignant disorders of the oral and oropharyngeal mucosa; terminology, classification and present concepts of management. Oral Oncology. 2009; **45**(4-5):317-323. DOI: 10.1016/j.oraloncology.2008.05.016

[10] Kalmar JR. Advances in the detection and diagnosis of oral precancerous and cancerous lesions. Oral and Maxillofacial Surgery Clinics of North America. 2006;**18**:465-482. DOI: 10.1016/j.coms.2006.06.013

[11] Okamura T et al. Disordered arrangements of basal cells as a prognostic factor for oral epithelial dysplasia: A morphometric study of 96 cases. Oral Surgery, Oral Medicine, Oral Pathology, and Oral Radiology. 2016;**122**(3):355-361. DOI: 10.1016/j.oooo.2016.05.005

[12] Hwang JTK et al. Individualized five-year risk assessment for oral premalignant lesion progression to cancer. Oral Surgery, Oral Medicine, Oral Pathology, Oral Radiology. 2017 Mar;**123**(3):374-381. DOI: 10.1016/j.oooo.2016.11.004

[13] Sciubba JJ, Helman JI. Current management strategies for verucous hyperkeratosis and verrucous carcinoma. Oral and Maxillofacial Surgery Clinics of North America. 2013 Feb;**25**(1):77-82, vi. DOI: 10.1016/j.coms.2012.11.008

[14] Na B et al. Oral cancer development in patients with oral lichen planus. Journal of Oral Pathology & Medicine 1993 Oct;**22**(9):421-424

[15] Grimm M et al. Analysis of circulating CD14 D/CD16 D monocyte-derived macrophages (MDMs) in the peripheral blood of patients with oral squamous cell carcinoma. Oral Surgery, Oral Medicine, Oral Pathology, and Oral Radiology. 2016;**121**(3):301-306. DOI: 10.1016/j.oooo.2015.10.024

[16] Warnakulasuriya S. Causes of oral cancer—An appraisal of controversies. BDJ. 2009; **207**(10):471-475. DOI: 10.1038/sj.bdj.2009.1009.

[17] Ali J et al. Genetic etiology of oral cancer. Oral Oncology. 2017;**70**:23-28. DOI: 10.1016/j.oraloncology.2017.05.004

[18] Ko L et al. Advances in brief allelic imbalance on chromosome 3p in oral dysplastic lesions: An early event in oral Carcinogenesis. Cancer Research. 1996;**56**:1228-1232

[19] Woo S et al. Biological significance of 5-hydroxymethylcytosine in oral epithelial dysplasia and oral squamous cell carcinoma. Oral Surgery, Oral Medicine, Oral Pathology, Oral Radiology. 2018 Jan;**125**(1):59-73.e2. DOI: 10.1016/j.oooo.2017.06.006. Epub 2017 Jun 16

[20] Harrandah AM et al. MicroRNA-375 as a biomarker for malignant transformation in oral lesions. Oral Surgery, Oral Medicine, Oral Pathology, and Oral Radiology. 2016; **122**(6):743-752.e1. DOI: 10.1016/j.oooo.2016.07.022

[21] Karatas OF et al. MicroRNAs in human tongue squamous cell carcinoma: From pathogenesis to therapeutic implications. Oral Oncology. 2017;**67**:124-130. DOI: 10.1016/j.oraloncology.2017.02.015

[22] Mishra R et al. High expression of survivin and its splice variants survivin D Ex3 and survivin 2 B in oral cancers. Oral Surgery, Oral Medicine, Oral Pathology, and Oral Radiology. 2015;**120**(4):497-507. DOI: 10.1016/j.oooo.2015.06.027

[23] Zhang L et al. Effects of human dachshund homolog 1 on the proliferation, migration, and adhesion of squamous cell carcinoma of the tongue. Oral Surgery, Oral Medicine, Oral Pathology, and Oral Radiology. 2016;**121**(1):58-66. DOI: 10.1016/j.oooo.2015.08.021

[24] Ohashi Y, Kumagai K, Miyata Y. Overexpression of ErbB4 is an independent marker for lymph node metastasis in Japanese patients with oral squamous cell carcinoma. Oral Surgery, Oral Medicine, Oral Pathology, and Oral Radiology. 2016;**122**(3):313-321. DOI: 10.1016/j.oooo.2016.04.017

[25] Takes RP. Staging of the neck in patients with head and neck squamous cell cancer: Imaging techniques and biomarkers. Oral Oncology. 2004 Aug;**40**(7):656-667. DOI: 10.1016/j.oraloncology.2003.11.001

[26] Matsui T, Shigeta T, Umeda M. Vascular endothelial growth factor C (VEGF-C) expression predicts metastasis in tongue cancer. Oral Surgery, Oral Medicine, Oral Pathology, and Oral Radiology. 2015;**120**(4):436-442. DOI: 10.1016/j.oooo.2015.06.002

[27] Moriyama M et al. Immunohistochemical study of tumour angiogenesis in oral squamous cell carcinoma. Oral Oncology. 1997 Sep;**33**(5):369-374

[28] Hu L et al. Transforming growth factor-b 1 activates D Np63/c-Myc to promote oral squamous cell carcinoma. Oral Surgery, Oral Medicine, Oral Pathology, and Oral Radiology. 2016;**122**(4):460-482.e4. DOI: 10.1016/j.oooo.2016.05.018

[29] Yang J et al. Prognostic value of toll-like receptor 4 and nuclear factor-k Bp65 in oral squamous cell carcinoma patients. Oral Surgery, Oral Medicine, Oral Pathology, and Oral Radiology. 2016;**122**(6):753-764.e1. DOI: 10.1016/j.oooo.2016.08.002

[30] Sakamoto T et al. Critical roles of Wnt5a – Ror2 signalling in aggressiveness of tongue squamous cell carcinoma and production of matrix metalloproteinase-2 via D Np63 b-mediated epithelial–mesenchymal transition. Oral Oncology. 2017;**69**:15-25. DOI: 10.1016/j.oraloncology.2017.03.019

[31] Takes RP. Staging of the neck in patients with head and neck squamous cell cancer: Imaging techniques and biomarkers. Oral Oncology. 2004 Aug;**40**(7):656-67. DOI: 10.1016/j.oraloncology.2003.11.001

[32] Scully C, Porter S. Oral Cancer Toolbox. BMJ. 2000;**321**:97-100

[33] Olshan A et al. Mouthwash use and cancer of the head and neck: A pooled analysis from the International Head and Neck Cancer Epidemiology Consortium (INHANCE). European Journal of Cancer Prevention. 2016 Jul;**25**(4):344-348. DOI: 10.1097/CEJ.0000000000000179

[34] Mirghani H et al. Human papilloma virus testing in oropharyngeal squamous cell carcinoma: What the clinician should know. Oral Oncology. 2014 Jan;**50**(1):1-9. DOI: 10.1016/j.oraloncology.2013.10.008. Epub 2013 Oct 26

[35] Khanal S et al. Histologic variation in high grade oral epithelial dysplasia when associated with high-risk human papillomavirus. Oral Surgery, Oral Medicine, Oral Pathology, and Oral Radiology. 2017;**123**(5):566-585. DOI: 10.1016/j.oooo.2017.01.008

[36] Garcia de A et al. Human papillomavirus in carcinomas of the tongue: Clinical and prognostic implications. International Journal of Oral & Maxillofacial Surgery. 2014 Mar;**43**(3):274-280

[37] Jiang R et al. Oral dysplasia and squamous cell carcinoma: Correlation between increased expression of CD21, Epstein-Barr virus and CK19. Oral Oncology. 2012 Sep;**48**(9):836-841. DOI: 10.1016/j.oraloncology.2012.03.017. Epub 2012 Apr 16

[38] Shamaa AA et al. The significance of Epstein Barr Virus (EBV) & DNA Topoisomerase II alpha (DNA-Topo II alpha) immunoreactivity in normal oral mucosa, Oral Epithelial Dysplasia (OED) and Oral Squamous Cell Carcinoma (OSCC). Diagnostic Pathology. 2008;**3**:45. https://doi.org/10.1186/1746-1596-3-45

[39] Berkovits C et al. Analysis of oral yeast microflora in patients with oral squamous cell carcinoma. Springer Plus. 2016. DOI: 10.1186/s40064-016-2926-6

[40] Bakri MM et al. Revisiting the association between candidal infection and carcinoma, particularly oral squamous cell carcinoma Journal of Oral Microbiology. 2010;**2**. DOI: 10.3402/jom.v2i0.5780

[41] Alnuaimi AD et al. Oral Candida colonization in oral cancer patients and its relationship with traditional risk factors of oral cancer: A matched case-control study. Oral Oncology. 2015;**51**(2):139-145. DOI: 10.1016/j.oraloncology.2014.11.008

[42] Javed F, Warnakulasuriya S. Is there a relationship between periodontal disease and oral cancer? A systematic review of currently available evidence. Critical Reviews in Oncology/Haematology. 2015:1-9. DOI: 10.1016/j.critrevonc.2015.08.018

[43] Abdulkareem AA et al. Periodontal pathogens promote epithelial-mesenchymal transition in oral squamous carcinoma cells in vitro. Cell Adhesion & Migration. 2017 Sep;**5**: 1-11. DOI: 10.1080/19336918.2017.1322253

[44] Gallimidi AB et al. Nucleatum promote tumour progression in an oral-specific chemical carcinogenesis model. Oncotarget. 2015 Sep 8;**6**(26):22613-22623

[45] Carneiro J, Alcino L, Porter SR. Review oral manifestations of syphilis. Clinics (Sao Paulo). 2006 Apr;**61**(2):161-166. Epub 2006 Apr 25

[46] Dickenson AJ, Currie WJR, Avery BS. Screening for syphilis in patients with carcinoma of the tongue. British Journal of Oral and Maxillofacial Surgery. Oct 1995;(5):319-320

[47] Visscher D et al. Squamous cell carcinoma of the lower lip in renal transplant recipients: Report of 6 cases. International Journal of Oral and Maxillofacial Surgery. 1997;**26**:120

[48] Gaston NK et al. Increased prevalence of dysplastic and malignant lip lesions in renal-transplant recipients. New England Journal of Medicine. 1995:1052-1057

[49] Thomas DW et al. Systemic immunosuppression and oral malignancy: A report of a case and review of the literature. British Journal of Oral and Maxillofacial Surgery. 1993 Dec;**31**(6);391-393. https://doi.org/10.1016/0266-4356(93)90197-5

[50] Kaplan I et al. Clinicopathologic evaluation of malignancy adjacent to dental implants. Oral Surgery, Oral Medicine, Oral Pathology, and Oral Radiology. 2017;**123**(1):103-112. DOI: 10.1016/j.oooo.2016.08.023

[51] Salgado-Peralvo AO et al. Is there an association between dental implants and squamous cell carcinoma? British Dental Journal. 2016;**221**(10):645-649. DOI: 10.1038/sj.bdj.2016.863

[52] Li Y, Peng J, Li L. Coffee consumption associated with reduced risk of oral cancer: A meta-analysis. Oral Surgery, Oral Medicine, Oral Pathology, and Oral Radiology. 2016; **121**(4):381-389.e1. DOI: 10.1016/j.oooo.2015.12.006

[53] Wang W, Zhang W, Wu W. Association of tea consumption and the risk of oral cancer: A meta-analysis. Oral Oncology. 2014;**50**(4):276-281. DOI: 10.1016/j.oraloncology.2013.12.014

[54] Rennemo E et al. Reduced risk of head and neck second primary tumours after radiotherapy. Radiotherapy and Oncology. 2009;**93**(3):559-562. DOI: 10.1016/j.radonc.2009.08.005

[55] Tae S et al. Chronic, reactive conditions of the oral cavity simulating mucosal carcinomas B CT and MR imaging findings with pathologic correlation in five patients. Clinical Imaging. 2005 Nov-Dec;**29**(6):406-611. DOI: 10.1016/j.clinimag.2005.06.026

[56] Kalavrezos N, Scully C. Mouth cancer for clinicians part 7: Cancer diagnosis and pretreatment preparation. Dental Update. 2016 Jan-Feb;**43**(1):50-54, 57-60, 63-65

[57] Lestón JS, Dios PD. Diagnostic clinical aids in oral cancer. Oral Oncology. 2010;**46**(6):418-422. DOI: 10.1016/j.oraloncology.2010.03.006

[58] Hiroshi Kurita KK. Vital staining with iodine solution in delineating the border of oral dysplastic lesions. Oral Surgery, Oral Medicine, Oral Pathology, Oral Radiology, and Endodontology. 1996 Mar;**81**(3):275-280

[59] Awan KH, Morgan PR, Warnakulasuriya S. Evaluation of an autofluorescence based imaging system (VELscope™) in the detection of oral potentially malignant dis orders and benign keratoses. Oral Oncology. 2011;**47**(4):274-277. DOI: 10.1016/j.oraloncology.2011.02.001

[60] El Hallani S et al. Ex vivo confocal imaging with contrast agents for the detection of oral potentially malignant lesions. Oral Oncology. 2013;**49**(6):582-590. DOI: 10.1016/j.oraloncology.2013.01.009

[61] Maurer K et al. Oral brush biopsy analysis by MALDI-ToF mass spectrometry for early cancer diagnosis. Oral Oncology. 2013;**49**(2):152-156. DOI: 10.1016/j.oraloncology.2012.08.012

[62] Toepker M et al. Can dual-energy CT improve the assessment of tumour margins in oral cancer? Oral Oncology. 2014;**50**(3):221-227. DOI: 10.1016/j.oraloncology.2013.12.001

[63] Payne KFB et al. The role of diffusion-weighted magnetic resonance imaging in the diagnosis, lymph node staging and assessment of treatment response of head and neck cancer. International Journal of Oral & Maxillofacial Surgery. International Association of Oral and Maxillofacial Surgery. 2015;**44**(1):1-7. DOI: 10.1016/j.ijom.2014.09.008

[64] Ouyang T, Iv BFB. Advances in head and neck imaging. Oral and Maxillofacial Surgery Clinics of NA. 2010;**22**(1):107-115. DOI: 10.1016/j.coms.2009.10.002

[65] Hass HG et al. DNA ploidy, proliferative capacity and intratumoral heterogeneity in primary and recurrent head and neck squamous cell carcinomas (HNSCC)—Potential implications for clinical management and treatment decisions. Oral Oncology. 2008 Jan;**44**(1):78-85. Epub 2007 Mar 9. DOI: 10.1016/j.oraloncology.2006.12.013

[66] Elimairi I et al. Oral paraneoplastic melanosis (OPM) as a rare presentation of neoplastic and non-neoplastic disease. Oral Surgery, Oral Medicine, Oral Pathology, and Oral Radiology. 2017;**124**(3):e198. DOI: 10.1016/j.oooo.2017.05.501

[67] Slater LJ. Odontogenic malignancies. Oral and Maxillofacial Surgery Clinics of North America. 2004;**16**(3):409-424

[68] Kamal M, Kaur P, Gupta R, Gupta S, Singh S. Mandibular plasmacytoma of jaw—A case report. Journal of Clinical and Diagnostic Research. 2014;**8**(8):20-21

[69] Shah A, Latoo S, Ahmad I. In: Gupta A. editor. Multiple Myeloma and Dentistry, Multiple Myeloma—An Overview. InTech; 2012. ISBN: 978-953-307-768-0. Available from: http://www.intechopen.com/books/multiple-myeloma-an-overview/multiple-myeloma-and-dentistry

[70] Berenice F, Gil D. Oral Kaposi's sarcoma in immunosuppressed patients—Report of cases. The South Brazilian Dentistry Journal RSBO (Online). 2013;**10**(1):89-95

[71] Douglas JL, Gustin JK, Moses AV, Dezube BJ, Pantanowitz L. Kaposi sarcoma pathogenesis: A triad of viral infection, oncogenesis and chronic inflammation. Translational Biomedicine. 2010;**1**(2). pii: 172

[72] Margaix-muñoz M, Bagán J, Poveda-roda R. Ewing sarcoma of the oral cavity. A review. 2017;**9**(2)

[73] Feller L, Khammissa RAG, Lemmer J. A review of the Aetiopathogenesis and clinical and Histopathological features of oral mucosal melanoma. Scientific World Journal. 2017;**2017**:1-7

[74] Arvind Babu RS, Ramana Reddy BV, Anuradha CH. Histogenetic concepts, terminology and categorization of biphasic tumours of the oral and maxillofacial region. Journal of Clinical and Diagnostic Research. 2014;**8**(2):266-270

Chapter 6

Thyroid Nodules in Diagnostic Pathology: From Classic Concepts to Innovations

Ilze Fridrihsone, Ilze Strumfa, Boriss Strumfs, Andrejs Vanags, Dainis Balodis, Arvids Jakovlevs, Arnis Abolins and Janis Gardovskis

Additional information is available at the end of the chapter

http://dx.doi.org/10.5772/intechopen.77117

Abstract

Thyroid nodules are frequent in general population, found in 3.7–7% of people by palpation and 42–67% by ultrasonography (US). The differential diagnosis ranges from papillary (PC), follicular (FC) and medullary (MC) carcinomas to follicular adenoma (FA) and colloid goitre. Cancer risk in thyroid nodules varies: 5% in masses found by palpation, 1.6–15% by US, 3.9–11.3% by computed tomography (CT), 5–6% by magnetic resonance imaging (MRI) and 30–50% by positron emission tomography (PET). The final diagnosis depends on fine needle aspiration (FNA) findings and histopathology. The recent WHO classification (2017) is based on classic morphology, including assessment of invasion and nuclei. New entities are defined to designate tumours with doubtful invasion or controversial nuclear features. By immunohistochemistry, PC expresses HBME-1, TROP-2, CITED1 and CK19. Notably, PC can stain for CD20. MC is recognised by neuroendocrine differentiation. To distinguish FA *vs.* FC, evaluation of HBME-1, p27 and galectin has been suggested. Regarding miRNAs, miR-146b, miR-222, miR-221 and miR-181b are upregulated, while miR-145, miR-451, miR-613 and miR-137 are downregulated in PC. FC features downregulated miR-199a-5p and upregulated miR-197 and miR-346. In MC, miR-21 and miR-129-5p are downregulated. In addition, increased systemic inflammatory reaction can be poor prognostic factor in thyroid cancer. The aim of this chapter is to review classic and innovative histopathology of thyroid nodules for diagnostic pathology practice and research in multidisciplinary thyroid teams.

Keywords: thyroid nodule, thyroid carcinoma, papillary carcinoma, follicular carcinoma, medullary carcinoma, histopathology, immunohistochemistry, miRNA, follicular adenoma

1. Introduction

Thyroid nodules represent an extremely frequent finding in the general population [1] and therefore enter the spectrum of the most common diagnostic dilemmas in endocrine surgery, cytology and surgical pathology. By palpation, such nodules can be found in 3.7–7% of general population, more frequently in females: 6.4% contrasting with 1.5% in males [2]. Three quarters of palpable nodules are solitary [3], raising increased suspicion of neoplasm. By ultrasonography (US), thyroid nodules can be disclosed even more frequently: in 42–67% of patients, and other radiological investigations also yield incidental nodules in a significant proportion of cases [2, 4–6] as shown in **Table 1**.

Malignant tumours do occur in thyroid albeit infrequently and can present as an incidentally found thyroid nodule (**Table 1**); therefore, reliable investigation is mandatory. The differential diagnostic approach should not be formal as evidence from a tertiary referral centre indicates that incidentally found thyroid carcinomas are even more frequently associated with lymphatic invasion and lymph node metastases [7]. However, the discrimination between malignant and benign thyroid masses can be difficult at all levels—radiology, fine needle aspiration (FNA) cytology and histopathology.

On the other hand, overdiagnosis of malignancy would lead to an unnecessary operation, carrying risks of complications. For instance, in a large group of 27,912 patients, included in the Surveillance, Epidemiology and End Results (SEER)-Medicare database, thyroid surgery-specific complications developed in 12.3% cases, while general postoperative complications were seen in 6.5% of patients [9]. Among the specific complications, hypoparathyroidism and vocal cord paralysis are the most frequent. The frequency of hypoparathyroidism in different studies ranges from 0.5 to 65% [10]. Transient hypoparathyroidism has been observed in 28.4–44.2% of patients, and 0.3–1.1% developed permanent hypoparathyroidism [11, 12]. After total thyroidectomy for well-differentiated thyroid carcinoma in 5670 SEER-Medicare patients (1991–2009), the frequency of unilateral *vs.* bilateral vocal cord paralysis was 8.2 *vs.* 1.3% [13]. Postoperative hematoma develops in 0.1–1% of patients and can lead to airway compression [14]. In addition, lifelong thyroid replacement treatment [15] is unavoidable after thyroidectomy. Psychological concerns and additional financial burden must be considered as well.

Evaluation method of the thyroid gland	Frequency of thyroid nodule, %	Cancer risk in the identified nodule, %	References
Palpation	3.7–7	5	[2]
Ultrasonography	42–67	1.6–15	[2, 8]
Computed tomography	16	3.9–11.3	[2]
Magnetic resonance imaging	4.5–5.1	5–6	[4–6]
Positron emission tomography	1.6 (for solitary pattern)	30–50 34.8 in meta-analysis	[2]

Table 1. Frequency of thyroid nodule and risk of malignancy by the method of investigation.

The rate of surgical complications is decreasing [13] due to novel approaches including continuous intraoperative neuromonitoring [10, 16, 17], novel haemostatic equipment, e.g., advanced bipolar electrocautery, ultrasound or hybrid devices and haemostatic agents for use close to vulnerable structures [14]; evaluation of surgeons' experience [18] and implementation of carbon nanoparticles to identify parathyroid glands [12, 19]. However, unnecessary surgery must be avoided. This, in turn, places greater demands on preoperative diagnostics, including immunohistochemical and/or molecular evaluation within the frames of multidisciplinary approach. Thus, the aim of this literature review is to summarise the present evidence in diagnostic pathology of thyroid nodules for the needs of practising pathologists as well as other colleagues working in multidisciplinary thyroid teams.

2. Epidemiology of thyroid carcinoma

The global incidence of thyroid cancer in 2012 was estimated as 6.1 per 100,000 women and 1.9 per 100,000 men. The gender-specific mortality rates were assessed as 0.6 and 0.3 per 100,000 respectively [20]. Generally, the epidemiology of thyroid carcinoma is characterised by growing incidence, decreasing global mortality and predominance of papillary carcinoma (PC). PC constitutes 65–93% of thyroid carcinomas [21, 22], while follicular carcinoma (FC) is responsible for 6–10% of thyroid carcinoma cases [21, 23]. Medullary carcinoma (MC) accounts for 2–5% of thyroid carcinomas [21, 24].

The incidence of thyroid cancer is growing in most countries and in both genders [20, 25], e.g., increasing from 4.9 to 14.3 per 100,000 individuals in USA over time period between 1975 and 2009 [26]. In the time period between 2000 and 2010, thyroid cancer-induced mortality in males has decreased in most European countries. However, it has increased significantly in Moldova (for 49.9%), Latvia (26.2%) and Portugal (15.7%). Regarding Americas, significant increase in mortality was seen in Costa Rica (66.9%), Uruguay (47.9%) and Ecuador (36.3%), while moderate – in USA (8.1%). New Zealand has also experienced increase in thyroid cancer-induced male mortality (14.5%). Regarding females, mortality from thyroid cancer has increased in Greece (13.3%), Colombia and Ecuador (both 17.8%), USA (6.8%) and Australia (14.0%). The 2008–2012 mortality levels were highest in Latvia, Estonia, Hungary, Moldova and Israel for males and in Ecuador, Colombia, Israel, Mexico and Latvia for females [20].

The growing incidence of thyroid carcinoma parallels increasing frequency of PC [26] and especially papillary microcarcinoma. Therefore, part of the scientific world considers the increase in incidence as the result of better diagnostics, yielding more incident nodules and enabling evaluation by US and biopsy even in as small lesions as measuring 2 mm in diameter. However, SEER-based data have clearly disclosed increased incidence of large PC as well. This corroborates the opinion that incidence growth purely reflects better diagnostics and incidental findings [2] and suggests true growth of incidence. In addition, incidental thyroid nodules are less frequently reported in clinical practice than in research. In a large retrospective analysis of 97,908 radiological reports, carried out in Chicago, USA, such nodules were noted in 0.4%, including 0.14% of computed tomography (CT), 0.64% of magnetic resonance imaging (MRI), 0.36% positron emission tomography (PET) scans and 6.59% US examinations. In contrast, on dedicated review, nodules were found in 10% of CT scans [27].

The reporting pattern is highly variable, depending both on nodule size and radiologist's specialisation [28]. Thus, the real input of incidental nodules in the growing incidence may be moderate.

The true increase of the incidence of thyroid carcinoma can be attributed to several risk factors, including changes in iodine supplement [25], adiposity [29, 30], oestrogens [31, 32], parity [33, 34], pregnancy-related increases in TSH levels [25], ionising radiation [35], and chemicals, e.g., polybrominated diphenyl ethers that are or have been used as flame retardants [25].

Many authors accentuate the gap between stable death rates and increasing numbers of new thyroid carcinoma cases suggesting "overestimation" of thyroid cancer [15], mainly small indolent PCs [20]. Existence of self-limiting thyroid cancers has been hypothesised based on: (1) lack of mortality reduction by surgery for papillary microcarcinoma; (2) low growth rate of papillary microcarcinoma and (3) high prevalence of papillary microcarcinoma in young people, contrasting with higher mortality in middle-aged patients. The consequences of this point of view include the conclusion that "the early detection of self-limiting cancers results in over-diagnosis" [36]. Possibly, most patients may not need treatment but those with high-risk disease must be promptly distinguished [20].

3. Radiological evaluation of a thyroid nodule

Neck US is the essential method in thyroid evaluation [37]. It can be both the starting point disclosing an incidental nodule and a reliable source of significant information for the final diagnosis. Thyroid nodule can be identified if US is performed for palpable neck mass, lymphadenopathy, suspected parathyroid or vascular pathology. The yield of thyroid nodules in such patients is 42–67%. In patients evaluated by cervical US for parathyroid disease, thyroid nodules are found in 20–56%, and the frequency of cancer in these lesions is 2–6%. By carotid artery duplex US, thyroid nodules have occasionally been more frequent (28%) than significant carotid stenosis (13%); the frequency of cancer in these nodules was 7.4%. The benefits of US include exact size measurements and possibility to disclose the features of malignant growth: hypoechoic nodule with irregular borders, central hypervascularity, presence of microcalcifications and elongated shape being taller than wide. US-guided FNA should be performed if the nodule exceeds the size of 1 cm or has additional worrisome features. Cancer risk in an incidental thyroid nodule, found by US, is 15% (not counting papillary microcarcinoma), being three times higher than in palpable nodule [2].

The innovations in ultrasonography include contrast-enhanced ultrasonography, elastography and superb microvascular imaging [1, 38, 39].

Computed tomography has a limited role in thyroid pathology. It is more informative in the beginning of the diagnostic way and in special situations. CT can provide the first evidence of thyroid nodule. In patients undergoing radiological examination for non-thyroid disease, cervical and thoracic CT yields thyroid nodules in up to 16% of cases. The risk of malignancy in CT-detected nodule ranges between 3.9 and 11.3%. Several pitfalls limit the informativity of CT in thyroid disease. These include the assessment of nodule size, number of lesions and risk of cancer. In studies comparing CT, US and postoperative findings, CT was shown to be less informative than US although both methods correlated with the findings in resected tissues. The size is the only reliable predictor of malignancy in CT, while presence of microcalcifications and attenuation in Hounsfield units are not specific. Because of these limitations, thyroid CT should be followed by US. CT can be useful in the further assessment of advanced cases to detect retrosternal spread, invasion into trachea and/or large vessels, metastases and recurrence in the site of operation, lymph nodes or distant tissue [2, 40].

Positron emission tomography usually is not included in the primary evaluation of thyroid. However, PET is increasingly performed for surveillance and staging of other malignant tumours. Occasionally, increased uptake in the thyroid has been noted in these patients. PET-positivity in the thyroid can manifest as diffuse uptake throughout the whole gland or as a solitary focus. The diffuse pattern is characteristic for Hashimoto thyroiditis or Graves' disease and carries low risk of malignancy: 4.4% comparable with 5% risk in palpable nodules. In contrast, solitary focus is a rare but worrisome finding: it is seen only in 1.6% of examined patients but the risk of malignant tumour reaches 30–50% (34.8% in a meta-analysis) as described by Wilhelm [2]. Therefore, US and FNA of a PET-positive focus are suggested regardless of size [2].

4. Histology and immunohistochemistry: From classics to innovations

4.1. Follicular adenoma

Follicular adenoma (FA) is defined as a benign, encapsulated, non-invasive thyroid tumour differentiating towards follicular epithelium and lacking the nuclear features of papillary thyroid carcinoma.

By autopsy findings, FAs have been reported in 3–5% of adults. Not surprisingly, this frequency is close to the prevalence of palpable solitary thyroid nodules. The known risk factors of FA include radiation exposure, especially in childhood and adolescence, and lack of iodine. Radiation exposure can cause FA after prolonged latent period (10–50 years), and the relative risk can reach 15. The role of iodine deficiency has been substantiated on more frequent findings of palpable thyroid nodules in areas of low iodine consumption. Although a fraction of such nodules will represent true FA, endemic sporadic goitre is classically triggered by iodine deficiency. Regarding hereditary factors, FAs are more frequent in patients having Cowden syndrome or familial adenomatous polyposis [3].

On US, FA represents a solid, well-demarcated, hypo- or isoechoic homogeneous mass. On radionuclide scan, most FAs are "cold" nodules, although "hot" adenomas are possible and can be associated by clinical hyperthyroidism [3].

FNA specimens from FA are characterised by high cellularity, rich presence of follicular cells, including microfollicles, and scant colloid. Macrofollicular FAs yield more colloid and monolayered sheets of epithelium. Inflammation, PC-type nuclei or psammoma bodies are absent. On FNA, differential diagnosis with follicular carcinoma is impossible as this would request identification of invasive growth. In addition, colloid-rich cytological specimens are similar to hyperplastic nodules [3].

Grossly, FAs are solitary, rounded, grey, whitish, tan or brown masses with smooth outline, contrasting with normal surrounding thyroid tissues. Microscopic structure is variable, but several key features are observed: (1) origin from follicular epithelium, mostly reflected in the follicular architecture; (2) structural difference from surrounding tissues; (3) presence of complete fibrous capsule; (4) lack of invasion; (5) lack of PC nuclear features and (6) lack of neuroendocrine differentiation. The architecture can be follicular (normo-, micro- or macro-), solid or trabecular. The cells are cuboidal or polygonal but can be cylindrical in "hot" adenomas. Cytoplasm is easily seen, eosinophilic or light. Nuclei are round, smooth, uniform, with evenly distributed, moderately dark chromatin. Mitoses are rare. Although stroma is usually scant, it can be more abundant in some tumours, exhibiting oedema, myxoid structure, haemorrhage, fibrosis and hyaline change as well as calcification. In distinction from hyperplastic nodule, solitary occurrence, presence of capsule and difference from surrounding thyroid tissues are helpful. In differential diagnosis with follicular carcinoma, lack of capsular and vascular invasion is the central criterion [3, 41].

FA has multiple histological variants including FA with papillary hyperplasia, lipoadenoma, FA with bizarre nuclei, signet ring cell FA, clear cell FA and spindle cell FA [3, 42].

4.2. Papillary thyroid carcinoma

Papillary carcinoma is a well-differentiated malignant thyroid tumour characterised by (1) origin from/differentiation towards follicular epithelium and (2) diagnostic nuclear features [22].

PC is the leading histological type of thyroid carcinomas, thus the risk factors are in line with the general risk factors of thyroid cancer, comprising ionising radiation, oestrogens, obesity, diabetes mellitus and ingestion of nitrates via food [22]. In contrast with FC, high iodine intake increases the risk of PC. Thus, iodine supplementation decreases the FC incidence and increases the PC occurrence. Despite higher PC frequency, the epidemiological change might be considered beneficial due to the favourable prognosis of papillary carcinoma.

On US examination, PC is hypo- or isoechoic, solid or cystic, irregularly shaped nodule that is taller than wide, contains microcalcifications and features disorganised vascular supply. By scintigraphy, papillary carcinomas mostly are "cold" [22].

By FNA, high cellularity is characteristic. Architecturally, papillae or monolayer sheets can be observed. Psammoma bodies are present. The cells are tall, showing visible cytoplasm. Nuclear changes are the most characteristic and diagnostically most important findings. These include thickened nuclear membranes and chromatin clearing, nuclear grooves and pseudoinclusions. The colloid can be either watery or thick, so-called ropy colloid. It might be more difficult to recognise the follicular variant and columnar variant having scarce nuclear features. Multiple nuclear inclusions can be seen in tall cell variant resulting in "soap bubble" appearance of the nuclei. Squamous metaplasia is possible in diffuse sclerosing variant; however, typical nuclear features are also present [22].

Grossly, PC is seen as a white, hard mass with irregular outline. Cystic change can be present while necrosis (in the absence of FNA history that might induce vascular collapse) is not characteristic and might indicate transformation to more aggressive tumour [22].

http://dx.doi.org/10.5772/intechopen.77117

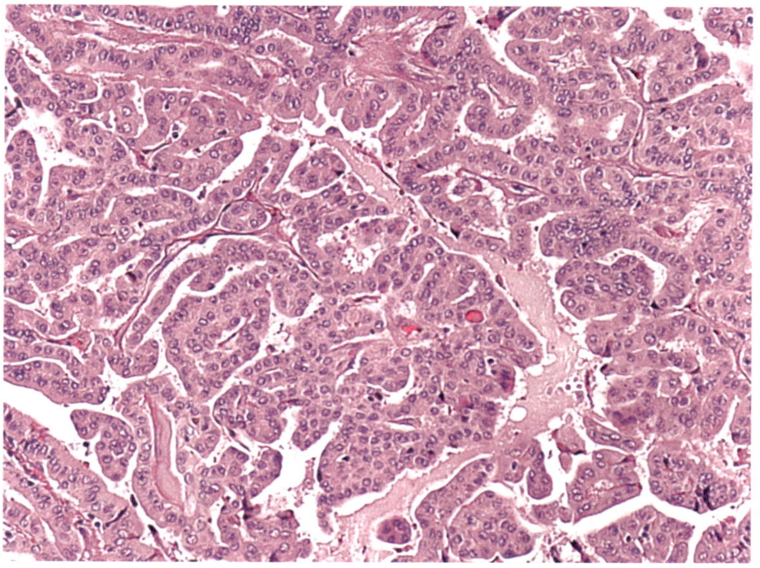

Figure 1. Papillary thyroid carcinoma. Note the characteristic architecture and nuclear features. Haematoxylin-eosin, original magnification 200×.

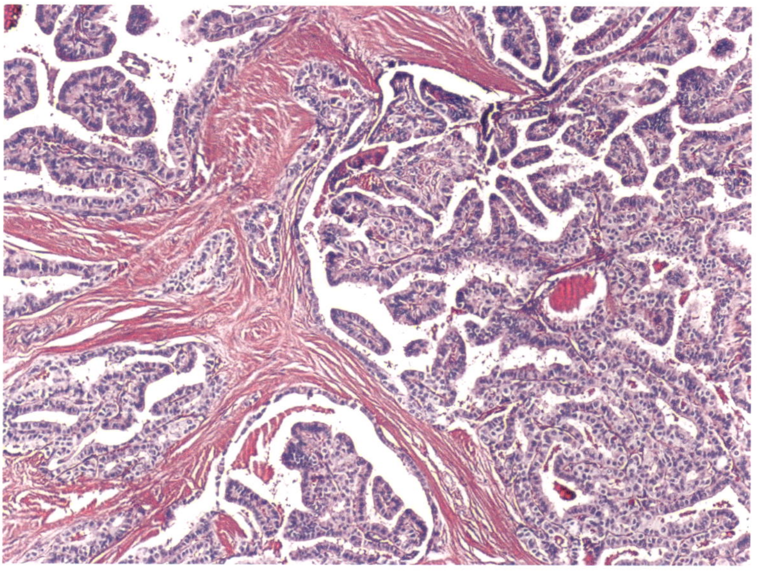

Figure 2. Stromal desmoplasia in papillary carcinoma. Haematoxylin-eosin, original magnification 100×.

Microscopically, PC is characterised by papillary architecture (**Figure 1**) and the diagnostic nuclear features. The papillae show significant variability between tumours, being straight or branched, loosely or tightly packed, long or short. Cystic or follicular foci are frequent. Solid and trabecular architecture can occur as well. Nuclei are enlarged, overlapping, elongated, characterised by membrane irregularity and optically empty "ground

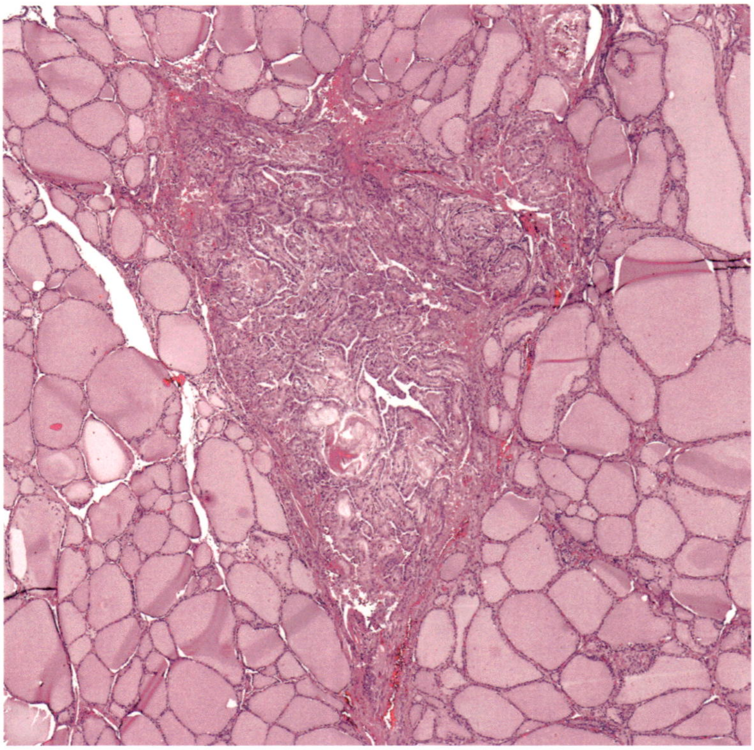

Figure 3. Papillary microcarcinoma in thyroid tissues. Haematoxylin-eosin, original magnification 50×.

glass" appearance. The "ground glass" appearance is very helpful in diagnostic evaluation of formalin-fixed, paraffin-embedded tissues. However, it is not seen in frozen sections compromising intraoperative assessment. The nuclear contour irregularity is seen as nuclear pseudoinclusions (of cytoplasm) and longitudinal grooves. Mitoses are rare. Psammoma bodies, present in 50% of cases, are small, rounded, laminated calcifications in stroma or lymphatic channels but not in colloid. Squamous metaplasia can be present. Stroma (**Figure 2**) is well developed [22, 41].

The histological variants of PC include papillary microcarcinoma (smaller than 1 cm; see **Figure 3**), encapsulated, follicular, diffuse sclerosing, tall cell, columnar cell, cribriform morular, hobnail, solid, oncocytic, spindle cell, clear cell and Warthin-like variants as well as PC with fibromatosis-like stroma [22, 43]. Carcinomas showing true papillary architecture are dominated by *BRAF* (*V600E*) mutations, while tumours holding follicular architecture mostly carry *RAS* mutations [44].

4.3. Follicular carcinoma

Follicular carcinoma is a malignant thyroid epithelial tumour characterised by follicular differentiation, invasive growth morphologically reflected in the invasion through capsule or into blood vessels and absence of the nuclear features of papillary carcinoma [23].

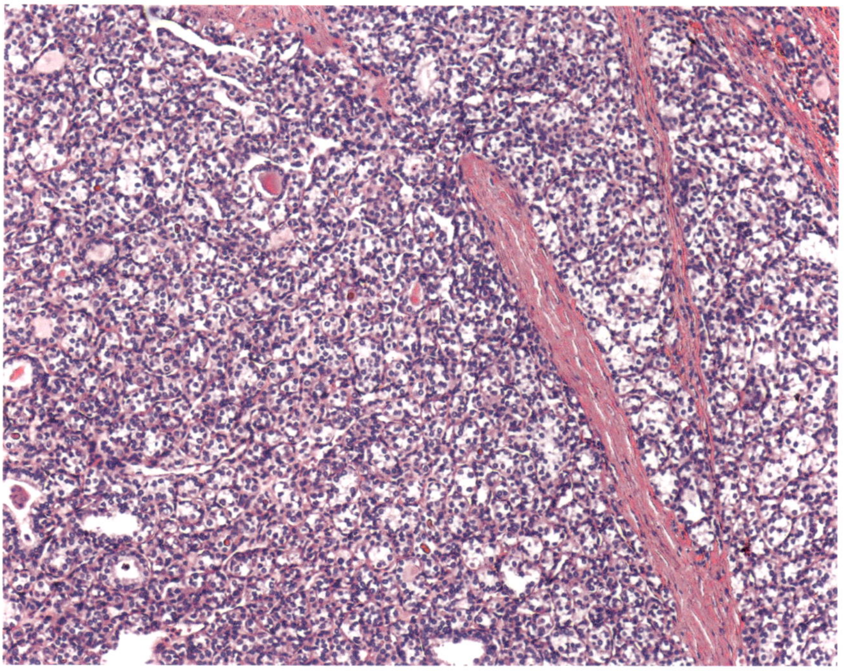

Figure 4. Follicular thyroid carcinoma. Note the invasion through the capsule. Haematoxylin-eosin, original magnification 200×.

The risk factors include low iodine supply and ionising irradiation although the association with radiation is weaker than for PC [23]. By FNA, FC cannot be distinguished from FA. Grossly, FCs are solid masses. Occasionally, the capsules seem thicker than in FA. Rarely, invasion through the capsule or into extrathyroid tissues is grossly evident.

Microscopically, the tumour is characterised by follicular architecture. By definition, there are no nuclear features that would define PC. The distinction from FA requires identification of invasion that can manifest as either minimal or wide capsular invasion (**Figure 4**) or angioinvasion (**Figure 5**). Minimal invasion is defined as focal, but unequivocal invasive growth that penetrates the full thickness of capsule. Irregular outline of the inner surface of the capsule or tumour cell groups within the capsule are insufficient for diagnosis. FC also must be strictly distinguished from artefacts such as surgery- or FNA-induced capsular lesions or curling of the tumour in the edges of tissue block. Vascular invasion must be assessed only in the capsule or extratumourally, not in the middle of the mass. To distinguish angioinvasion from artefactual contamination of blood vessels by tumour cells, e.g., during grossing, any intravascular tumour cell group should be qualified as an evidence of invasion only if the tumour tissues are adherent to blood vessel walls, covered by either endothelium or fibrin, or thrombus [23, 41]. Morphologic variants are rare, including clear cell [23], signet ring cell [45], microcystic and spindle cell variants, FC with fat cells and FC with glomeruloid pattern [23]. Mucinous variant has been reported [46].

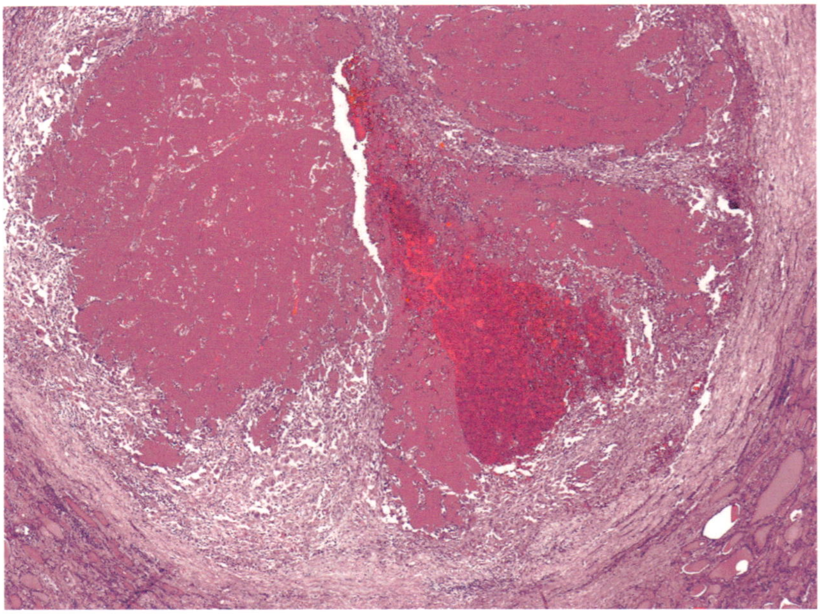

Figure 5. Invasion of a follicular thyroid carcinoma in a large blood vessel. Haematoxylin-eosin, original magnification 50×.

4.4. Follicular tumours with controversial morphology

In the recent WHO classification (2017), certain new entities have been defined to classify thyroid tumours with controversial morphological appearance, doubtful invasion or questionable nuclear features [47].

Follicular-patterned tumours showing unequivocal capsular or vascular invasion are designated as (1) invasive follicular variant of PC, if the nuclei show typical structure of PC; (2) well differentiated thyroid carcinoma, not otherwise specified, if the nuclear features are controversial; and (3) FC, if the nuclei lack any traits of PC.

Tumours that are definitely non-invasive are designated FA, if the nuclear structure is certainly of non-papillary type. Otherwise, the diagnosis of non-invasive follicular thyroid neoplasm with papillary-like nuclear features is issued [48]. Finally, tumours with questionable invasion are designated either follicular tumours of uncertain malignant potential if the nuclei are of non-papillary type or well-differentiated tumour of uncertain malignant potential in all other cases.

These new entities provide pathologists with the long-awaited benefit of accurate diagnosis. However, the biological potential of these groups still remains to be assessed. Generally, the risk of recurrence or metastasis is low, but exceptions still have been reported [47].

4.5. Medullary carcinoma

Medullary carcinoma is a malignant thyroid tumour showing C-cell differentiation [49].

MC is characterised by high fraction of hereditary tumours, reaching up to 30%. In contrast, the risk factors of sporadic MC are almost unknown [49]. Activating *RET* mutations are present in 40% of sporadic MC and over 90% of hereditary cases, mostly with almost complete penetrance [50].

FNA shows round, ovoid or spindle cells. Eccentric position of the nucleus can impart plasmacytoid appearance. Chromatin is granular. Amyloid can be present in the specimen. Despite immunohistochemical investigation, diagnosis is correctly recognised in only 46.1% of cases [49]. In our experience, systematic immunohistochemical approach to all thyroid tumours lacking typical papillary type nuclei is helpful to avoid a diagnostic mistake. Serum calcitonin level would also disclose the diagnosis in most cases.

Grossly, the lesions are grey to yellow, featuring different consistencies. Bilateral and multicentric growth is characteristic for inherited tumours [49]. Microscopic picture can be very confusing due to the variety of histological patterns—MC is the "great mimic." However, the immunophenotype is distinctive in most cases, and the presence of local amyloidosis can significantly guide the diagnostic thinking, enhancing the suspicion for MC.

The architecture of MC is solid, trabecular, lobular or insular. The cells are polygonal, plasmacytoid, spindled or show mixed morphology. Nuclei are round, with coarse chromatin and small nucleoli. The cytoplasm ranges from eosinophilic to amphophilic. Calcitonin-containing amyloid is present in 90% of cases. The presence of nuclear pseudoinclusions and rare psammoma bodies can be misleading. Hereditary tumours are accompanied by C cell hyperplasia. The variants include papillary, follicular, spindle cell, giant cell, clear cell, oncocytic, melanotic, squamous, amphicrine, paraganglioma-like, angiosarcoma-like, encapsulated and small cell MC [41, 49, 51]. MC is characterised by neuroendocrine phenotype, and immunohistochemistry for chromogranin A, calcitonin or related peptides, and carcinoembryonic antigen is highly advised to confirm the diagnosis.

4.6. Metastases to the thyroid gland

Metastases of extrathyroid tumours (MTS) to the thyroid gland are rare. In FNA cytology, MTS constituted 2.2% of cases [52]. However, they are encountered in diagnostic surgical pathology as well as in FNA cytology and can have very misleading morphology. The authors of a recent clinical series have reported on 32 such cases [53]. Among these patients, lung was the most frequent site of primary tumour (14/32), followed by renal and gastrointestinal cancers at equal frequency of 5/32. Interestingly, MTS affecting the thyroid were diagnosed over wide time range, from manifestation simultaneously with the primary cancer to delayed presentation 16 years after the initial diagnosis. Although thyroidectomy was not considered in patients affected by an aggressive cancer at high stage, it still has been performed in 34.5% of patients having secondary thyroid tumour, and the longest survival was 7 years [53].

The spectrum of MTS differs between hospitals, e.g., renal cell carcinoma (48.1%), colorectal (10.4%), pulmonary (8.3%) and breast carcinoma (7.8%) as well as sarcomas (4.0%) were observed in German series [54]. Wide scope of primary tumours was disclosed in cytologically investigated cases, including pulmonary (6/20), gastrointestinal, breast (each 5/20), laryngeal (3/20) and renal cell (1/20) carcinoma [52].

In the largest series of secondary thyroid tumours, comprising 97 patients who underwent FNA in Mayo Clinic, lung and kidney were the most frequent primary sites (22% each), followed by head and neck cancer (12%) as reported by Hegerova et al. [55]. Similarly to the observations by Zhang et al. [53], prolonged survival was seen in some patients, reaching 228 months (median, 20 months). Thyroid resection was not infrequent: it was performed in 41/97 patients reaching survival of 30 months (range, 3–171 months), while the median survival in non-operated patients was 12 months (range, 1–228 months). The difference was statistically insignificant [55].

Metastases of cutaneous or uveal melanomas have been reported and can present a major diagnostic problem considering that melanoma is another "great mimic" in pathology [56].

4.7. Immunohistochemistry of thyroid neoplasms

Although in most cases routine stains are sufficient for correct classification of a thyroid nodule, ancillary methods are occasionally necessary. Immunohistochemistry (IHC) is a well-known, easily applicable technology, nowadays complemented with automatization and digital evaluation. The expenses are moderate, making IHC a widely available approach. It benefits from high accuracy of antigen-antibody reaction and visual evaluation of the positive targets resulting in correct interpretation.

In thyroid pathology, several antigen groups have been explored. Antigens that are specific for thyroid follicular cells (thyroglobulin, TTF-1) are useful to identify the follicular origin of a neoplasm. Expression is observed in PC [22], FA [3] and FC [23] as well as in Hurtle cell tumours. MC is negative for thyroglobulin but can exhibit a weak staining for TTF-1 [49], although controversial opinions have been expressed. A possible pitfall is nuclear expression of TTF-1 in non-squamous lung cancer MTS (adenocarcinoma, small cell carcinoma, large cell carcinoma). Lung cancer lacks thyroglobulin but can express surfactant apoprotein A (adenocarcinoma), napsin A (adenocarcinoma; however, positive reaction in thyroid cancers has been reported) or neuroendocrine markers (small cell carcinoma and large cell neuroendocrine carcinoma).

Neuroendocrine markers (chromogranin A, synaptophysin) along with calcitonin are characteristic of MC [49] and C-cell hyperplasia. PC and FA are negative for chromogranin A, other neuroendocrine markers and calcitonin [3, 22].

Membrane proteins, including HBME-1, TROP-2, beta-galactoside-binding protein family galectins and glypicans (one of the two protein families within heparin sulphate proteoglycan class), are helpful in PC diagnostics. Cytoskeleton composition by certain intermediate filaments (cytokeratin (CK) 19, vimentin) also shows correlation with specific pathological processes. Proliferation activity in carcinomas is generally higher than in benign nodules but the levels in differentiated cancers are too low to set a reliable diagnostic threshold. Nevertheless, proteins that are involved in cell cycle regulation and apoptosis have been evaluated in thyroid pathology.

Hector Battifora mesothelial epitope, widely known by the abbreviation HBME-1, is a membranous antigen, located on microvilli of benign and malignant mesothelial cells [57, 58]. In the thyroid, intense HBME-1 expression is characteristic for PC [22, 59]. Membranous pattern is the most specific [22]. Diffuse and intense membranous expression is strongly supportive for PC diagnosis [60]. A fraction of FC is positive [23], but reactivity in FA is considered rare [3].

The reported expression rate of HBME-1 in PC ranges between 73.8% [61], 75.9% [62], 85.0% [63] and 96.1% [64]. Higher frequency has been found in classic PC, e.g., ranging between 95.9 and 100% in contrast to 45.0–81.1% in follicular variants [61, 65]. However, some authors report close findings in classic or follicular variant. Thus, in a large IHC study of 127 thyroid tumours, including 49 classic PCs, 29 cases of follicular variant of papillary carcinoma (FVPC) and 49 FAs, HBME-1 was expressed in 88% of classic PC and 86% cases of FVPC, contrasting with 4% in FA [60].

The expression of HBME-1 in PC differs from surrounding benign thyroid tissues [66]. In a large study of 177 thyroid glands (including 53 PCs, 11 FVPC cases, 13 FCs and 100 benign thyroids), HBME-1 was expressed in 74% of PC and 89% of FVPC, but was not found (0%) in Graves' disease or nodular colloid goitre [67]. Prasad et al. also confirmed the absence of HBME-1 in Graves' disease and normal thyroid but experienced a single case (1%) of positive nodular goitre [63]. Higher expression rate in benign thyroid tissues (7.0%) has been reported by Nasr et al. [64]. The HMBE-1 reactivity in follicular neoplasms also differs remarkably between studies: 17% [67] *vs.* 26.7% [62] *vs.* 50.0% [63] *vs.* 85.7% [68] of FC and 4% [60] *vs.* 10% [63] *vs.* 11% [67] *vs.* 14.8% [62] *vs.* 64% [68] of FA.

The differences might be attributable to the evaluation (pattern: membranous only *vs.* membranous and cytoplasmic), cut-off threshold, selection of primary antibodies, epitope retrieval, dilution, incubation temperature and incubation time. Thus, although HBME-1 is among the most sensitive and specific antigens in the PC diagnostics [61] and has been included in most diagnostic panels [58] for PC or thyroid cancer (predominated by PC), controversies remain.

Few, but promising reports are available on human trophoblast cell surface antigen TROP-2 in PC, which seems to be a reliable marker in histology and cytology, holding high specificity and sensitivity [61, 69–71]. The TROP-2 protein is absent from MC, follicular tumours and non-neoplastic thyroid tissue [70, 71], while it is present in 82.5% of PC. The limits of the marker include diagnostics of follicular variant which shows less frequent and focal staining. Nevertheless, the presence of 10% positive cells in a tumour indicates PC, and the heterogeneity is sufficiently low to apply TROP-2 IHC on FNA specimens [70]. Again, data on expression frequency are variable. Thus, in a recent study, TROP-2 was found in between 90.0 and 95.3% PC and 70.0% follicular variants [71]. However, other research groups have described significantly less frequent reactivity: 50% [61].

CITED1 (the abbreviation for CREB (cAMP-response element-binding protein)/ p300 interacting transactivator with glutamic acid/ aspartic acid-rich carboxy-terminal domain 1) protein, encoded by *CITED1* gene, acts as transcriptional activator. The expression pattern is nuclear and cytoplasmic [63]. CITED1 enhances SMAD-mediated transcription by strengthening the interaction between DNA, transcription factors and coactivators (SMAD is an acronym coined by the fusion of names for the *Sma* gene in *Caenorhabditis elegans* and the "mothers against decapentaplegic" *Mad* gene in *Drosophila*). In association with SMAD pathway, CITED1 promotes signalling via transforming growth factor beta (TGF-beta) molecular pathway. CITED1 also stabilises interaction between oestrogen receptors and histone acetyltransferase, enhancing oestrogen-dependent gene expression, and associates with chromatin in oestrogen-dependent way.

CITED1 is expressed in PC [22]. Some authors consider it useful in differential diagnostics between PC, including follicular variant, and FA [43, 72] as expression of CITED1 in FA is considered rare [3]. However, CITED1 has been found in both benign and malignant pathologies. Thus, in a large study of 177 thyroid glands (including 53 PCs, 11 FVPC cases, 13 FCs and 100 benign thyroids), CITED1 was expressed not only in 98% of PC, 100% of FVPC, and 86% of FC but also in 89% of Graves' disease cases, 79% of nodular colloid goitre and 80% of FA [67]. More promising data were obtained in another large IHC study of 127 thyroid tumours, including 49 classic PCs, 29 FVPC cases and 49 FAs. CITED1 was expressed in 90% of classic PC and 83% FVPC cases, contrasting with 16% of FA [60]. Similarly, CITED1 was expressed in 93% of PC, 25% of FC, 10% of FA and 8% of nodular goitre, but it was not found in normal thyroid glands and Graves' disease cases [63]. Among 215 formalin-fixed, paraffin-embedded thyroid specimens, CITED1 was expressed in 87% PC and 50% FC while only 10% of FA and 24% of nodular goitre were positive, but cases of Graves' disease and normal thyroid were invariably negative [63].

CITED1 expression is dependent on technological issues. One of the described rabbit antibodies has been associated with increased background to such a degree that interferes with reliable evaluation. However, another rabbit antibody has also been considered as having lower sensitivity and specificity in comparison with HBME-1 and CK19 [60].

Knowing the role of CITED1 in PC and the epidemiological evidence of higher incidence in females, it is not surprising to find expression of oestrogen and progesterone receptors in papillary carcinoma. Expression of oestrogen receptor alpha and progesterone receptor has been reported in 19% and 38.7–57% of PC cases, correspondingly [73, 74].

Galectins represent a family of proteins that are defined by the capacity to bind beta-galactoside carbohydrates. Galectins are located in cell nuclei, cytoplasm or extracellular space. Galectins are classified into dimeric, tandem and chimera classes. Dimeric galectins, e.g., galectin-1, are simple homodimers. Tandem galectins contain one or more carbohydrate recognition domains in a single peptide chain. Chimeric class, represented only by galectin-3, has long non-lectin domain. Such chimeric molecule can exist as a monomer (at low concentration) or form multimers (at high concentration), if up to five monomers are linked by non-lectin domain. The physiologic effects are different: while monomers inhibit adhesion by blocking adhesion proteins, pentamers create intercellular bridges or link cells and extracellular matrix.

Expression of galectin-3 in FA is rare [3]. Galectin-3 is more frequently seen in malignant thyroid tumours [75], and this finding has strong pathogenetic basis. Knockdown or antagonists of galectin-3 suppress the migratory capacity of PC cells. Galectin-3 is upregulated by hypoxia-inducible factor (HIF)-1 [76]. In PC, the expression rate has been estimated as 64.7% [65] *vs.* 69% [61] *vs.* 92% [67] or even 100% [77]. Lower rate has been reported in follicular variant: 33 *vs.* 92% in classic cases [67]. However, some authors describe close findings in classic or follicular variant. Thus, in a large IHC study of 127 thyroid tumours, including 49 classic PCs, 29 FVPC cases and 49 FAs, galectin-3 was expressed in 96% of classic PC and 90% FVPC cases, contrasting with 18% in FA [60]. The expression frequency reached 97% in a small mixed group of carcinomas, comprising 22 PCs (16 classic and six FVPC cases), 3 FCs, 5 MCs and a single Hurtle cell carcinoma [75]. Among 13 FCs, the expression rate was 33% [67]. The staining pattern should be both nuclear and cytoplasmic [22]. Notably, benign reactive epithelial and inflammatory cells in Hashimoto thyroiditis can express galectin-3 [22, 60]. No expression was found in Graves' disease and nodular colloid goitre by Liu et al. [67]. However, other research groups have noted the presence of galectin-3 in 55% of nodular goitre and 7% of Graves' diseases cases while normal thyroid tissues were invariably negative [63]. FA has been described as negative [67] or occasionally (18%) positive [60]. In general, galectin-3 has been found in 10% [63] *vs.* 30% [75] *vs.* 43% [77] FA, more frequently (80%) in Hurtle cell adenomas [77]. Even the authors reporting less frequent positivity in FA, consider galectin-3 as a second-line marker due to lower specificity and sensitivity [60].

Along with CK19 and galectin-3, galectin-1 is more frequently expressed in PC than in FA. Loss of galectin-1 activity suppresses proliferation, migration and invasion [78]. In cell cultures, galectin-1 has been evaluated as the target for vectorised contrast agent, bearing peptide-conjugated ultrasmall superparamagnetic iron oxide particles for MRI [79].

Glypicans along with syndecans represent the major protein families of heparin sulphate proteoglycans. Glypicans are involved in developmental processes as well as regulation of cell signalling by Wnt and Hedgehog pathways. Glypican-3 is more frequently expressed in malignant thyroid tumours. Among 17 FA, the expression rate was 24%. Higher positivity rate (81%) was observed in a small mixed group of carcinomas, comprising 22 PCs, 3 FCs, 5 MCs and one case of Hurtle cell carcinoma [75]. In a larger group, glypican-3 was found in 100% (20/20) of FC and 70% (48/69) of PC [80].

PCs are characterised by upregulation of CD44 and its ligand osteopontin. Expression of osteopontin in PC is statistically significantly higher than normal thyroid tissue, colloid goitre and FA. In addition, the presence and intensity of osteopontin expression correlates with proliferation activity [81], capacity to invade and occurrence of adverse prognostic factors such as lymph node metastases and large size of the tumour [82]. Expression of osteopontin is found in 83.3% of PC, 70.0% of benign thyroid nodules and 50.0% of normal thyroid tissues [83]. Limited amount of information is available on osteopontin in FC, but upregulation has been shown in dogs [84]. In MC, osteopontin is expressed in 78.4% of cases and shows association with good prognostic features [85]. The levels of bone sialoprotein are increased in PC. Thus, expression of bone sialoprotein is found in 87.9% of PC, 55.0% of benign thyroid nodules and 42.5% of normal thyroid tissues [83]. PC is characterised by statistically significant cytoplasmic and membranous upregulation of vitamin D receptor in comparison to non-neoplastic thyroid tissues. Cancer cells also possess vitamin-D inactivating 24-hydroxylase but not activating enzyme, namely, 1-alpha-hydroxylase. Overexpression of 24-hydroxylase is associated with extrathyroid invasion and lymph node metastases [74].

Regarding CD44 variant 6 protein, the positive cell fraction in PC constitutes 80.3% while only 37.1% of cells in benign thyroid nodules and 22.9% of normal thyroid epithelial cells are positive [86]. Stem cell marker CD44 is involved in epithelial-mesenchymal transition (EMT), characterised by loss of epithelial markers, e.g., E-cadherin, and appearance of mesenchymal proteins, e.g., vimentin. Expression of vimentin was found in 53.8% of PC and 75% of FC [87]. PCs feature loss of E-cadherin in contrast to surrounding benign thyroid tissues. Nevertheless, E-cadherin along with CD56 is upregulated in FA [88]. However, if cancer is assessed separately, not within the context with surrounding tissues, E-cadherin is still retained. Thus, expression of E-cadherin was found in 84.6% of PC and 75% of FC [87].

Claudins are another class of EMT-associated proteins [89]. In FC, transmembrane tight junction protein claudin is dislocated from membrane to nucleus. Switch in subcellular compartmentalisation leads to increased proliferation, invasion and migration [90].

Among cytokeratins, CK19 has attracted attention. Intense expression of CK19 is considered a valuable diagnostic marker in PC [91], although it is the least specific marker of malignancy [22, 59]. In PC, reported expression rates of CK19 range between 45.6% [65], 83.3% [61] and 84.6% [87]. Expression of CK19 was found in 25% of FC [87]. However, in a large study of 177 thyroids (including 53 PCs, 11 FVPC cases, 13 FCs and 100 benign glands), CK19 was found in 78% of PC, 22% of follicular variants, but was absent from FC, FA, Graves' disease cases and nodular colloid goitre [67]. Promising data were obtained in another IHC study of 127 thyroid tumours, including 49 classic PC, 29 FVPC cases and 49 FA. CK19 was expressed in 100% of classic PC and 90% FVPC cases, contrasting with 14% of FA [60]. Nevertheless, in another study, CK19 was found in 100% PC and even 68.4% of benign thyroid tissues [64]. In a significant cohort of 215 thyroids, CK19 was expressed in 72% of PC, 50% of FC, 5% of FA, 31% of nodular goitre, 0% of Graves' disease and 7% of normal thyroids [63].

CK19 is considered to have high sensitivity but lower specificity in the differential diagnosis between PC and FA. However, not mere presence but also the intensity and distribution of expression matters. The expression in PC tends to be strong and diffuse while FA shows focal and weaker staining. The expression in nodular hyperplasia and normal thyroid tissues also tends to be focal and weak [60]. The comparison between nodule and surrounding tissues would be important. In addition, PC is positive for pancytokeratin and CK7, but negative for CK20—a fact that in rare circumstances is helpful to distinguish between PC and thyroid metastases from a colorectal adenocarcinoma known to express CK20 [22].

In contrast with surrounding benign thyroid tissues, PC is characterised by downregulation of CD56 [59, 88]. The frequency of CD56 loss ranges from 93.9% in classic PC to 73.3% in FVPC cases [65]. In contrast, CD56 is upregulated in FA [88].

Regarding regulation of cell proliferation and apoptosis, PC is associated with increased expression of phosphorylated histone H3 and cyclin D1. Metastatic PCs exhibit upregulated caspase-3 and loss of anti-apoptotic Bcl-2 [92]. Cyclins A and B1 are found in PC as well [93]. Autophagy-related protein Beclin-1 is more frequently seen in thyroid carcinomas. The expression rate is 98.9% in PC and 57.1% in FC while only 21.4% of FAs are positive for Beclin-1. The level of Beclin-1 correlates with proliferation activity by Ki-67 [68]. Survivin is more frequently expressed in carcinomas and is associated with the biological potential of the neoplasm [94]. Cytoplasmic location of p27 has been observed in PC [95], and p27 along with galectin has been advised to discriminate between FA and FC [96].

PC is characterised by complete or almost complete loss of c-kit/CD117 protein contrasting with benign thyroid nodules and normal follicular epithelium [97].

Aberrant membranous expression of CD20 has recently been reported in PC [98, 99]. In a small group of PC, expression was found in 5/22 (23%) tumours [99]. The findings were confirmed in a large cohort of 538 PCs [98] disclosing reactivity in 10% of cases. Although CD20 was associated with less aggressive morphological features of PC, expression in anaplastic

Panel	Aim	Cohort	References
HBME-1, galectin-3, CK19	FVPC *vs.* FA	157 thyroid tumours, 5 normal glands	[72]
HBME-1, galectin-3, CITED1	FVPC *vs.* FA	157 thyroid tumours, 5 normal glands	[72]
HBME-1, CK19 Second line: CITED1, galectin-3	PC *vs.* FA	127 thyroid tumours: 49 classic PC, 29 FVPC, 49 FA	[60]
HBME-1, CK19	PC *vs.* benign thyroid tissues	51 PC, 57 benign cases	[64]

HBME, Hector Battifora mesothelial epitope; CK, cytokeratin; CITED1, the abbreviation for CREB (cAMP-response element-binding protein)/ p300 interacting transactivator with glutamic acid/ aspartic acid-rich carboxy-terminal domain 1; FVPC, follicular variant of papillary carcinoma; FA, follicular adenoma and PC, papillary carcinoma.

Table 2. Immunohistochemical panels in the diagnostics of thyroid nodules.

thyroid cancers was observed with similar frequency (6–20%) as in PC. FAs (47) were negative. Positivity of CD20 was not associated with other B lymphocyte lineage markers as CD79alpha or PAX5 [98] but was confirmed by two different clones of primary antibody [99].

Neuroendocrine differentiation is the hallmark of MC that is positive for chromogranin A in 92.9% of cases [100]. Regarding the other regional causes of chromogranin A-positive mass lesions, parathyroid adenoma (that can occur intrathyroidally) and parathyroid hyperplasia are characterised by expression rates of 28/28 and 7/8 [100]. IHC panels should include calcitonin and carcinoembryonic antigen CEA (to identify MC with 100% specificity, as reported by Wuertz et al.) and parathyroid hormone that is expressed in 72.2% parathyroid nodules [100].

In most MCs, calcitonin is present [101]. In the rare cases of non-secretory MC, IHC diagnosis is still possible by panel of calcitonin, CEA and chromogranin A [102]. Among 75 MC, calcitonin receptor was expressed in 82.7% of cases. It showed strong positive correlation with calcitonin ($p = 0.001$) and osteocalcin ($p = 0.009$) as reported by Cappagli et al. [103]. CEA expression is characteristic and is mostly widespread and moderate to strong by intensity [104]. Presence of CD56 has been reported [101].

Clusterin is another lineage-specific IHC marker, expressed in C cells, C cell hyperplasia and primary and metastatic MC. In addition, prognostic value of clusterin score has been reported, with inverse correlation between clusterin score and presence of lymph node metastases [105]. Survivin and X-linked inhibitor of apoptosis (XIAP) are expressed in C cells and MC and are associated with worse survival [106]. Expression of HIF-1alpha is another prognostic marker. Positive expression has been shown to be associated with worse 5-year survival and progression free survival [107]. Stem cell markers CD133 and CD44 are unfavourable prognostic predictors. Both CD133 and CD44 are independent factors associated with worse overall survival, while CD44 is also significantly associated with recurrence-free survival [108]. Expression of somatostatin receptors 2A and 5 correlates with advanced stages [109]. Heat shock proteins HSP70, HSP90 and GRP78 are upregulated in MC in comparison with normal thyroid tissues [110]. Upregulation of cancer/testis antigens is seen, contrasting with negative normal thyroid tissues and goitre as well as with rare expression in PC and FC. However, poorly differentiated and anaplastic carcinomas are also positive [111].

Recognising the diversity of thyroid nodules and variability of IHC data, panel diagnostics is advised (see examples in **Table 2**).

5. miRNAs in thyroid tumours

Biochemical and biological alterations of cancer cells are largely supported by non-coding RNA (ncRNA) dysregulation in the tumour. Non-coding RNAs lack an open-reading frame and do not have protein-coding ability. Based on the size of the functional RNA molecule, regulatory ncRNAs are classified as long ncRNAs and small ncRNAs or microRNAs [112]. MicroRNAs (miRNA) are small, evolutionary conserved, single-stranded, non-coding RNA molecules (approximately 22 nucleotides in length) that bind target mRNA to regulate gene expression [113, 114]. MicroRNAs are involved in various physiological and pathological functions, such as apoptosis, cell proliferation and differentiation, which indicate their functionality in carcinogenesis as tumour suppressor genes or oncogenes [115]. Up or downregulation of miRNA can influence the tumorigenic outcome depending on the role(s) of the target genes on vital signalling processes [116].

The most often upregulated miRNAs in PC are miR-146b, miR-222, miR-221 and miR-181b. Overexpressed miR-146b targets retinoic acid receptor beta (RARβ) and reduces expression of this gene leading to increased tumour aggressiveness and extrathyroidal invasion [117–120]. MiR-221 and miR-222 target tumour suppressor and cell cycle regulator p27. Reduced expression of p27 results in increased proliferation of tumour cells. These processes are related to aggressive behaviour of tumour, extrathyroidal invasion and spread to lymph nodes [117–120]. MiR-181b is also overexpressed in PC compared to normal thyroid tissue. MiR-181b inhibits expression of cylindromatosis *CYLD* gene, which acts as tumour suppressor and normally induces apoptosis [118, 121].

The most often downregulated miRNAs in PC are miR-145, miR-451, miR-613 and miR-137. MiR-145 acts as a tumour suppressor in thyroid cancer, and its downregulation enhances cancer growth via several pathways [118]. MiR-451 functions as a tumour suppressor by targeting the PI3/AKT pathway. Downregulation of miR-451a is associated with aggressive tumour course and the presence of extrathyroidal invasion [118, 120]. In PC, miR-613 is involved in cell proliferation and invasion [117, 118], but downregulated miR-137 leads to increased cellular proliferation, invasion and migration [118].

The miRNAs found in FC are also frequently present in other subtypes of thyroid cancer [120]. MiR-199a-5p is downregulated, but miR-197 and miR-346 are upregulated in FC resulting in increased cancer cell proliferation [118].

Many miRNAs have been found to be dysregulated in thyroid cancer, but only few miRNAs are exclusively associated with anaplastic thyroid cancer [118]. Loss of miR-200 expression in anaplastic carcinoma results in EMT that represses the epithelial features of cancer cells and disrupts the cell-cell adhesion mediated by loss of E-cadherin. This process enables cells to migrate and invade [116, 118, 120].

In MC, miR-21 is recently studied. It is downregulated, especially in the aggressive cases [120]. MiR-129-5p is significantly downregulated in MC compared to normal tissue leading to increased cellular invasion and migration [118].

6. Systemic inflammatory reaction in thyroid carcinoma patients

Systemic inflammatory response (SIR) is induced by different types of cancer [122, 123]. Interaction between the tumour and the host inflammatory response is crucial in cancer development [122, 124]. Many studies confirm the association between increased SIR and poor outcome in cancer patients [124, 125]. To evaluate SIR, different parameters are used: neutrophil-to-lymphocyte ratio (NLR), platelet-to-lymphocyte ratio (PLR), concentration of acute phase proteins, clotting factors and albumins, e.g., Glasgow Prognostic Score (GPS) and others [123, 126]. The role of SIR in thyroid cancer is still poorly understood. Authors of several studies have suggested that increased NLR is associated with larger tumour size and increased recurrence risk of thyroid cancer [127, 128].

7. Conclusions

In conclusion, thyroid nodules represent an important problem in endocrine surgery as a frequent finding inducing complicated differential diagnostics. In general population, such nodules are found in 3.7–7% by palpation and 42–67% by US. Cancer risk in thyroid nodule varies: 5% in masses found by palpation, 1.6–15% by US, 3.9–11.3% by CT, 5–6% by MRI and 30–50% by PET.

The epidemiological picture of thyroid carcinoma is characterised by growing incidence and stable or decreasing mortality, suggesting overtreatment of an indolent disease. However, mortality growth is seen in some countries, e.g., in Costa Rica (for 66.9%), Moldova (49.9%), Uruguay (47.9%), Latvia (26.2%), Ecuador (36.3%), New Zealand (14.5%) and Portugal (15.7%) for males and Colombia, Ecuador (both 17.8%) or Greece (13.3%) for females. In addition, SEER data disclose growing incidence of large carcinomas. Clinically, incidental thyroid nodules are reported less frequently than in dedicated research studies. Thus, true incidence growth can be related to risk factors such as changes in iodine supplementation, adiposity, oestrogens, parity, pregnancy-related increases in TSH levels, exposure to ionising radiation and chemicals, e.g., polybrominated diphenyl ethers, used as flame retardants.

The final diagnosis of thyroid tumours, dominated by benign follicular adenomas and malignant papillary, follicular and medullary carcinomas, depends on FNA and histopathology. Classic morphology, based on invasion and nuclear features, substantiates the diagnosis in most cases and represents the basis of WHO diagnostic criteria.

A significant innovation is the definition of new entities in the recent WHO classification to designate thyroid tumours with controversial morphological appearance, doubtful invasion or questionable nuclear features. Follicular tumours that definitely lack invasion but exhibit controversial nuclear structure are classified as non-invasive follicular thyroid neoplasm with papillary-like nuclear features. Follicular-patterned neoplasms with questionable invasion are called either follicular tumours of uncertain malignant potential if the nuclei are of non-papillary type or well-differentiated tumour of uncertain malignant potential in other cases. These new entities provide pathologists with the long-awaited benefit of accurate diagnosis.

Ancillary methods include the widely accessible immunohistochemistry and rapidly developing field of miRNA analysis. HBME-1, TROP-2, CITED1 and CK19 can be helpful in diagnostics of papillary carcinoma, while galectin-3 might serve as second-line marker. Expression of CD20 in PC has been recently reported. Distinction between FA and FC is difficult; HBME-1, p27 and galectin evaluation has been recommended. MC holds neuroendocrine differentiation.

Regarding miRNAs, PC is characterised by upregulation of miR-146b, miR-222, miR-221 and miR-181b and downregulation of miR-145, miR-451, miR-613 and miR-137. FC features downregulated miR-199a-5p and upregulated miR-197 and miR-346. In MC, miR-21 and miR-129-5p are downregulated.

Initial studies suggest that increased SIR can be poor prognostic factor in thyroid cancer.

Acknowledgements

The present work was supported by scientific project No. 1.1.1.2./VIAA/1/16/242 (BS).

Conflict of interest

The authors report no conflicts of interest to disclose.

Author details

Ilze Fridrihsone[1]*, Ilze Strumfa[1], Boriss Strumfs[2], Andrejs Vanags[3], Dainis Balodis[1], Arvids Jakovlevs[1], Arnis Abolins[1] and Janis Gardovskis[3]

*Address all correspondence to: Ilze.Fridrihsone@rsu.lv

1 Department of Pathology, Riga Stradins University, Riga, Latvia

2 Latvian Institute of Organic Synthesis, Riga, Latvia

3 Department of Surgery, Riga Stradins University, Riga, Latvia

References

[1] Ahn HS, Lee JB, Seo M, Park SH, Choi BI. Distinguishing benign from malignant thyroid nodules using thyroid ultrasonography: Utility of adding superb microvascular imaging

and elastography. La Radiologia Medica. 2018;**123**(4):260-270. DOI: 10.1007/s11547-017-0839-2 [Epub ahead of print]

[2] Wilhelm S. Evaluation of thyroid incidentaloma. The Surgical Clinics of North America. 2014;**94**(3):485-497. DOI: 10.1016/j.suc.2014.02.004

[3] Nikiforov YE, Baloch ZW, Belge G, Chan JKC, Derwahl KM, Evans HL, Fagin JA, Ghossein RA, Lloyd RV, Oriola J, Osamura RY, Paschke R, Sobrinho Simoes M. Follicular adenoma. In: Lloyd RV, Osamura RY, Kloppel G, Rosai J, editors. WHO Classification of Tumours of Endocrine Organs. 4th ed. Lyon: International Agency for Research on Cancer; 2017. pp. 69-72

[4] Choi N, Moon WJ, Kim HY, Roh HG, Choi JW. Thyroid incidentaloma detected by time-resolved magnetic resonance angiography at 3T: Prevalence and clinical significance. Korean Journal of Radiology. 2012;**13**(3):275-282. DOI: 10.3348/kjr.2012.13.3.275

[5] Lim HK, Park ST, Ha H, Choi SY. Thyroid nodules detected by contrast-enhanced magnetic resonance angiography: Prevalence and clinical significance. PLoS One. 2016;**11**(2): e0149811. DOI: 10.1371/journal.pone.0149811

[6] Kim K, Emoto N, Mishina M, Okada S, Isu T, Yoshida D, Kobayashi S, Teramoto A. Incidental detection of thyroid nodules at magnetic resonance imaging of the cervical spine. Neurologia Medico-Chirurgica (Tokyo). 2013;**53**(2):77-81. DOI: https://doi.org/10.2176/nmc.53.77

[7] Farra JC, Picado O, Liu S, Ouyang W, Teo R, Franco AM, Lew JI. Clinically significant cancer rates in incidentally discovered thyroid nodules by routine imaging. The Journal of Surgical Research. 2017;**219**:341-346. DOI: 10.1016/j.jss.2017.06.050

[8] Hoang JK, Nguyen XV. Understanding the risks and harms of management of incidental thyroid nodules: A review. JAMA Otolaryngology. Head & Neck Surgery. 2017; **143**(7):718-724. DOI: 10.1001/jamaoto.2017.0003

[9] Papaleontiou M, Hughes DT, Guo C, Banerjee M, Haymart MR. Population-based assessment of complications following surgery for thyroid cancer. The Journal of Clinical Endocrinology and Metabolism. 2017;**102**(7):2543-2551. DOI: 10.1210/jc.2017-00255

[10] Cannizzaro MA, Lo Bianco S, Picardo MC, Provenzano D, Buffone A. How to avoid and to manage post-operative complications in thyroid surgery. Updates in Surgery. 2017;**69**(2):211-215. DOI: 10.1007/s13304-017-0475-3

[11] Lee YS, Nam KH, Chung WY, Chang HS, Park CS. Postoperative complications of thyroid cancer in a single center experience. Journal of Korean Medical Science. 2010;**25**(4): 541-545. DOI: 10.3346/jkms.2010.25.4.541

[12] Su A, Wang B, Gong Y, Gong R, Li Z, Zhu J. Risk factors of hypoparathyroidism following total thyroidectomy with central lymph node dissection. Medicine (Baltimore). 2017; **96**(39):e8162. DOI: 10.1097/MD.0000000000008162

[13] Francis DO, Pearce EC, Ni S, Garrett CG, Penson DF. Epidemiology of vocal fold paralyses after total thyroidectomy for well-differentiated thyroid cancer in a Medicare population. Otolaryngology and Head and Neck Surgery. 2014;**150**(4):548-557. DOI: 10.1177/0194599814521381

[14] Materazzi G, Ambrosini CE, Fregoli L, De Napoli L, Frustaci G, Matteucci V, Papini P, Bakkar S, Miccoli P. Prevention and management of bleeding in thyroid surgery. Gland Surgery. 2017;**6**(5):510-515. DOI: 10.21037/gs.2017.06.14

[15] Brito JP, Morris JC, Montori VM. Thyroid cancer: Zealous imaging has increased detection and treatment of low risk tumours. British Medical Journal. 2013;**347**:f4706. DOI: 10.1136/bmj.f4706

[16] Schneider R, Machens A, Randolph GW, Kamani D, Lorenz K, Dralle H. Opportunities and challenges of intermittent and continuous intraoperative neural monitoring in thyroid surgery. Gland Surgery. 2017;**6**(5):537-545. DOI: 10.21037/gs.2017.06.08

[17] Yang S, Zhou L, Lu Z, Ma B, Ji Q, Wang Y. Systematic review with meta-analysis of intraoperative neuromonitoring during thyroidectomy. International Journal of Surgery. 2017;**39**:104-113. DOI: 10.1016/j.ijsu.2017.01.086

[18] Adam MA, Thomas S, Youngwirth L, Hyslop T, Reed SD, Scheri RP, Roman SA, Sosa JA. Is there a minimum number of thyroidectomies a surgeon should perform to optimize patient outcomes? Annals of Surgery. 2017;**265**(2):402-407. DOI: 10.1097/SLA.0000000000001688

[19] Huang K, Luo D, Huang M, Long M, Peng X, Li H. Protection of parathyroid function using carbon nanoparticles during thyroid surgery. Otolaryngology and Head and Neck Surgery. 2013;**149**(6):845-850. DOI: 10.1177/0194599813509779

[20] La Vecchia C, Malvezzi M, Bosetti C, Garavello W, Bertuccio P, Levi F, Negri E. Thyroid cancer mortality and incidence: A global overview. International Journal of Cancer. 2015;**136**(9):2187-2195. DOI: 10.1002/ijc.29251

[21] Lukas J, Drabek J, Lukas D, Dusek L, Gatek J. The epidemiology of thyroid cancer in the Czech Republic in comparison with other countries. Biomedical Papers of the Medical Faculty of the University Palacky, Olomouc, Czech Republic. 2013;**157**(3):266-275. DOI: 10.5507/bp.2012.086

[22] Rosai J, Albores Saavedra J, Asioli S, Baloch ZW, Bogdanova T, Chen H, DeLellis RA, Erickson LA, Fagin JA, Franssila KO, Giordano TJ, Hay ID, Katoh R, Lloyd RV, Mete O, Nikiforov YE, Piana S, Prasad ML, Sadow P, Schneider AB, Soares P, Sobrinho Simoes M, Vielh P, Wenig BM. Papillary thyroid carcinoma. In: Lloyd RV, Osamura RY, Kloppel G, Rosai J, editors. WHO Classification of Tumours of Endocrine Organs. 4th ed. Lyon: International Agency for Research on Cancer; 2017. pp. 81-91

[23] LiVolsi V, Abdulkader Nallib I, Baloch ZW, Bartolazzi A, Chan JKC, DeLellis RA, El Naggar AK, Eloy C, Eng C, Fagin JA, Ghossein RA, Giordano TJ, Kondo T, Lloyd RV, Mete O, Nikiforov YE, Nonaka D, Paschke R, Perren A, Rosai J, Sadow P, Schneider AB, Sobrinho Simoes M, Tallini G, Williams MD. Folicular thyroid carcinoma. In: Lloyd RV, Osamura RY, Kloppel G, Rosai J, editors. WHO Classification of Tumours of Endocrine Organs. 4th ed. Lyon: International Agency for Research on Cancer; 2017. pp. 92-95

[24] Tormey WP, Byrne B, Hill AD, Sherlock M, Thompson CJ. Should serum calcitonin be routinely measured in patients presenting with thyroid nodule? Minerva Endocrinologica. 2017;**42**(4):306-310. DOI: 10.23736/S0391-1977.17.02566-4

[25] Kilfoy BA, Zheng T, Holford TR, Han X, Ward MH, Sjodin A, Zhang Y, Bai Y, Zhu C, Guo GL, Rothman N, Zhang Y. International patterns and trends in thyroid cancer incidence, 1973-2002. Cancer Causes & Control. 2009;**20**(5):525-531. DOI: 10.1007/s10552-008-9260-4

[26] Davies L, Welch HG. Current thyroid cancer trends in the United States. JAMA Otolaryngology. Head & Neck Surgery. 2014;**140**(4):317-322. DOI: 10.1001/jamaoto.2014.1

[27] Uppal A, White MG, Nagar S, Aschebrook-Kilfoy B, Chang PJ, Angelos P, Kaplan EL, Grogan RH. Benign and malignant thyroid incidentalomas are rare in routine clinical practice: A review of 97,908 imaging studies. Cancer Epidemiology, Biomarkers & Prevention. 2015;**24**(9):1327-1331. DOI: 10.1158/1055-9965.EPI-15-0292

[28] Grady AT, Sosa JA, Tanpitukpongse TP, Choudhury KR, Gupta RT, Hoang JK. Radiology reports for incidental thyroid nodules on CT and MRI: High variability across subspecialties. AJNR. American Journal of Neuroradiology. 2015;**36**(2):397-402. DOI: 10.3174/ajnr.A4089

[29] Schmid D, Ricci C, Behrens G, Leitzmann MF. Adiposity and risk of thyroid cancer: A systematic review and meta-analysis. Obesity Reviews. 2015;**16**(12):1042-1054. DOI: 10.1111/obr.12321

[30] Colditz GA, Peterson LL. Obesity and cancer: Evidence, impact and future directions. Clinical Chemistry. 2018;**64**(1):154-162. DOI: 10.1373/clinchem.2017.277376

[31] Derwahl M, Nicula D. Estrogen and its role in thyroid cancer. Endocrine-Related Cancer. 2014;**21**(5):T273-T283. DOI: 10.1530/ERC-14-0053

[32] Rajoria S, Hanly E, Nicolini A, George AL, Geliebter J, Shin EJ, Suriano R, Carpi A, Tiwari RK. Interlinking of hypoxia and estrogen in thyroid cancer progression. Current Medicinal Chemistry. 2014;**21**(11):1351-1360. DOI : 10.2174/0929867321666131201142434

[33] Zhu J, Zhu X, Tu C, Li YY, Qian KQ, Jiang C, Feng TB, Li C, Liu GJ, Wu L. Parity and thyroid cancer risk: A meta-analysis of epidemiological studies. Cancer Medicine. 2016;**5**(4):739-752. DOI: 10.1002/cam4.604

[34] Zabuliene L, Jasilionis D, Miseikyte-Kaubriene E, Stukas R, Kaceniene A, Smailyte G. Parity and risk of thyroid cancer: A population-based study in Lithuania. Hormones & Cancer. 2017;**8**(5-6):325-329. DOI: 10.1007/s12672-017-0308-3

[35] Wartofsky L. Increasing world incidence of thyroid cancer: Increased detection or higher radiation exposure? Hormones (Athens, Greece). 2010;**9**(2):103-108

[36] Takano T. Natural history of thyroid cancer [review]. Endocrine Journal. 2017;**64**(3):237-244. DOI: 10.1507/endocrj.EJ17-0026

[37] Grani G, Lamartina L, Cantisani V, Maranghi M, Lucia P, Durante C. Interobserver agreement of various thyroid imaging reporting and data systems. Endocrine Connections. 2018;**7**(1):1-7. DOI: 10.1530/EC-17-0336

[38] Prieditis P, Radzina M, Strumfa I, Narbuts Z, Ozolins A, Vanags A, Gardovskis J. Diagnostic value of contrast-enhanced ultrasound evaluation of malignant and benign solitary thyroid nodules. Proceedings of the Latvian Academy of Sciences. Section B. 2016;**70**(1):1-6. DOI: 10.1515/prolas-2016-0001

[39] Lu R, Meng Y, Zhang Y, Zhao W, Wang X, Jin M, Guo R. Superb microvascular imaging (SMI) compared with conventional ultrasound for evaluating thyroid nodules. BMC Medical Imaging. 2017;**17**(1):65. DOI: 10.1186/s12880-017-0241-5

[40] Suh CH, Baek JH, Choi YJ, Lee JH. Performance of CT in the preoperative diagnosis of cervical lymph node metastasis in patients with papillary thyroid cancer: A systematic review and meta-analysis. AJNR. American Journal of Neuroradiology. 2017;**38**(1):154-161. DOI: 10.3174/ajnr.A4967

[41] Moghaddam PA, Virk R, Sakhdari A, Prasad ML, Cosar EF, Khan A. Five top stories in thyroid pathology. Archives of Pathology & Laboratory Medicine. 2016;**140**(2):158-170. DOI: 10.5858/arpa.2014-0468-RA

[42] Agaimy A, Hahn T, Schroeder J, Elhag A. Follicular thyroid adenoma dominated by spindle cells: Report of two unusual cases and literature review. International Journal of Clinical and Experimental Pathology. 2012;**5**(2):143-151

[43] Lloyd RV, Buehler D, Khanafshar E. Papillary thyroid carcinoma variants. Head and Neck Pathology. 2011;**5**(1):51-56. DOI: 10.1007/s12105-010-0236-9

[44] Giordano TJ. Follicular cell thyroid neoplasia: Insights from genomics and The Cancer Genome Atlas research network. Current Opinion in Oncology. 2016;**28**(1):1-4. DOI: 10.1097/CCO.0000000000000248

[45] Romero-Rojas AE, Diaz-Perez JA, Mastrodimos M, Chinchilla SI. Follicular thyroid carcinoma with signet ring cell morphology: Fine-needle aspiration cytology, histopathology, and immunohistochemistry. Endocrine Pathology. 2013;**24**(4):239-245. DOI: 10.1007/s12022-013-9271-x

[46] Squillaci S, Pitino A, Spairani C, Ferrari M, Carlon E, Cosimi MF. Mucinous variant of follicular carcinoma of the thyroid gland: Case report and review of the literature. International Journal of Surgical Pathology. 2016;**24**(2):170-176. DOI: 10.1177/1066896915617026

[47] Chan JKC, Nikiforov YE, Tallini G. Other encapsulated follicular-patterned thyroid tumours. In: Lloyd RV, Osamura RY, Kloppel G, Rosai J, editors. WHO Classification of Tumours of Endocrine Organs. 4th ed. Lyon: International Agency for Research on Cancer; 2017. pp. 75-80

[48] Range DE, Jiang XS. An update on noninvasive follicular thyroid neoplasm with papillary-like nuclear features. Current Opinion in Oncology. 2018;**30**(1):1-7. DOI: 10.1097/CCO.0000000000000416

[49] DeLellis RA, Al Ghuzlan A, Albores Saavedra J, Baloch ZW, Basolo F, Elisei R, Kaserer K, LiVolsi V, Matias-Guiu X, Mete O, Moley JF, Nikiforov YE, Nose V, Pinto AE. Medullary thyroid carcinoma. In: Lloyd RV, Osamura RY, Kloppel G, Rosai J, editors. WHO Classification of Tumours of Endocrine Organs. 4th ed. Lyon: International Agency for Research on Cancer; 2017. pp. 108-113

[50] Chu YH, Lloyd RV. Medullary thyroid carcinoma: Recent advances including microRNA expression. Endocrine Pathology. 2016;**27**(4):312-324. DOI: 10.1007/s12022-016-9449-0

[51] Baloch ZW, LiVolsi VA. C-cells and their associated lesions and conditions: A pathologists perspective. Turkish Journal of Pathology. 2015;**31**(Suppl 1):60-79. DOI: 10.5146/tjpath.2015.01315

[52] Rossi ED, Martini M, Straccia P, Gerhard R, Evangelista A, Pontecorvi A, Fadda G, Maria Larocca L, Schmitt F. Is thyroid gland only a "land" for primary malignancies? Role of morphology and immunocytochemistry. Diagnostic Cytopathology. 2015;**43**(5):374-380. DOI: 10.1002/dc.23241

[53] Zhang L, Liu Y, Li X, Gao W, Zheng C. Metastases to the thyroid gland: A report of 32 cases in PUMCH. Medicine (Baltimore). 2017;**96**(36):e7927. DOI: 10.1097/MD.0000000000007927

[54] Schmid KW. Lymph node and distant metastases of thyroid gland cancer. Metastases in the thyroid glands (Article in German). Der Pathologe. 2015;**36**(Suppl 2):171-175. DOI: 10.1007/s00292-015-0071-6

[55] Hegerova L, Griebeler ML, Reynolds JP, Henry MR, Gharib H. Metastasis to the thyroid gland: Report of a large series from the Mayo Clinic. American Journal of Clinical Oncology. 2015;**38**(4):338-342. DOI: 10.1097/COC.0b013e31829d1d09

[56] Collins DC, Yela R, Horgan N, Power DG. A rare thyroid metastasis from uveal melanoma and response to immunotherapy agents. Case Reports in Oncological Medicine. 2016;**2016**:6564094. DOI: 10.1155/2016/6564094

[57] Mase T, Funahashi H, Koshikawa T, Imai T, Nara Y, Tanaka Y, Nakao A. HBME-1 immunostaining in thyroid tumors especially in follicular neoplasm. Endocrine Journal. 2003;**50**(2):173-177. DOI: https://doi.org/10.1507/endocrj.50.173

[58] Arcolia V, Journe F, Renaud F, Leteurtre E, Gabius HJ, Remmelink M, Saussez S. Combina tion of galectin-3, CK19 and HBME-1 immunostaining improves the diagnosis of thyroid cancer. Oncology Letters. 2017;**14**(4):4183-4189. DOI: 10.3892/ol.2017.6719

[59] Erdogan-Durmus S, Ozcan D, Yarikkaya E, Kurt A, Arslan A. CD56, HBME-1 and cytokeratin 19 expressions in papillary thyroid carcinoma and nodular thyroid lesions. Journal of Research in Medical Sciences. 2016;**21**:49. DOI: 10.4103/1735-1995.183986

[60] Scognamiglio T, Hyjek E, Kao J, Chen YT. Diagnostic usefulness of HBME1, galectin-3, CK19, and CITED1 and evaluation of their expression in encapsulated lesions with questionable features of papillary thyroid carcinoma. American Journal of Clinical Pathology. 2006;**126**(5):700-708. DOI: 10.1309/044V-86JN-2W3C-N5YB

[61] Murtezaoglu AR, Gucer H. Diagnostic value of TROP-2 expression in papillary thyroid carcinoma and comparison with HBME-1, galectin-3 and cytokeratin 19. Polish Journal of Pathology. 2017;**68**(1):1-10. DOI: 10.5114/pjp.2017.67610

[62] Dunderovic D, Lipkovski JM, Boricic I, Soldatovic I, Bozic V, Cvejic D, Tatic S. Defining the value of CD56, CK19, Galectin-3 and HBME-1 in diagnosis of follicular cell derived lesions of thyroid with systematic review of literature. Diagnostic Pathology. 2015;**10**:196. DOI: 10.1186/s13000-015-0428-4

[63] Prasad ML, Pellegata NS, Huang Y, Nagaraja HN, de la Chapelle A, Kloos RT. Galectin-3, fibronectin-1, CITED-1, HBME1 and cytokeratin-19 immunohistochemistry is useful for the diagnosis of thyroid tumors. Modern Pathology. 2005;**18**(1):48-57. DOI: 10.1038/modpathol.3800235

[64] Nasr MR, Mukhopadhyay S, Zhang S, Katzenstein AL. Immunohistochemical markers in diagnosis of papillary thyroid carcinoma: Utility of HBME1 combined with CK19 immunostaining. Modern Pathology. 2006;**19**(12):1631-1637. DOI: 10.1038/modpathol.3800705

[65] Nechifor-Boila A, Borda A, Sassolas G, Hafdi-Nejjari Z, Borson-Chazot F, Lifante JC, Sturm N, Laverriere MH, Berger N, Decaussin-Petrucci M. Immunohistochemical markers in the diagnosis of papillary thyroid carcinomas: The promising role of combined immunostaining using HBME-1 and CD56. Pathology, Research and Practice. 2013;**209**(9):585-592. DOI: 10.1016/j.prp.2013.06.012

[66] Ozolins A, Narbuts Z, Strumfa I, Volanska G, Gardovskis J. Diagnostic utility of immunohistochemical panel in various thyroid pathologies. Langenbeck's Archives of Surgery. 2010;**395**(7):885-891. DOI: 10.1007/s00423-010-0690-6

[67] Liu YY, Morreau H, Kievit J, Romijn JA, Carrasco N, Smit JW. Combined immunostaining with galectin-3, fibronectin-1, CITED-1, Hector Battifora mesothelial-1, cytokeratin-19, peroxisome proliferator-activated receptor-{gamma}, and sodium/iodide symporter antibodies for the differential diagnosis of non-medullary thyroid carcinoma. European Journal of Endocrinology. 2008;**158**(3):375-384. DOI: 10.1530/EJE-07-0492

[68] Yesil C, Kandemir O, Haksever H, Dabakoglu T. Is BECLIN-1 immunoreactivity more effective than HBME-1 in diagnosis of papillary thyroid cancer? Acta Chirurgica Belgica. 2015;**115**(4):299-305. DOI: 10.1080/00015458.2015.11681116

[69] Addati T, Achille G, Centrone M, Petroni S, Popescu O, Russo S, Grammatica L, Simone G. TROP-2 expression in papillary thyroid cancer: A preliminary cyto-histological study. Cytopathology. 2015;**26**(5):303-311. DOI: 10.1111/cyt.12196

[70] Bychkov A, Sampatanukul P, Shuangshoti S, Keelawat S. TROP-2 immunohistochemistry: A highly accurate method in the differential diagnosis of papillary thyroid carcinoma. Pathology. 2016;**48**(5):425-433. DOI: 10.1016/j.pathol.2016.04.002

[71] Simms A, Jacob RP, Cohen C, Siddiqui MT. TROP-2 expression in papillary thyroid carcinoma: Potential diagnostic utility. Diagnostic Cytopathology. 2016;**44**(1):26-31. DOI: 10.1002/dc.23382

[72] Nakamura N, Erickson LA, Jin L, Kajita S, Zhang H, Qian X, Rumilla K, Lloyd RV. Immu nohistochemical separation of follicular variant of papillary thyroid carcinoma from follicular adenoma. Endocrine Pathology. 2006;**17**(3):213-223

[73] Eldien MMS, Abdou AG, Rageh T, Abdelrazek E, Elkholy E. Immunohistochemical expression of ER-α and PR in papillary thyroid carcinoma. Ecancermedicalscience. 2017;**11**:748. DOI: 10.3332/ecancer.2017.748

[74] Yavropoulou MP, Panagiotou G, Topouridou K, Karayannopoulou G, Koletsa T, Zarampoukas T, Goropoulos A, Chatzaki E, Yovos JG, Pazaitou-Panayiotou K. Vitamin

D receptor and progesterone receptor protein and gene expression in papillary thyroid carcinomas: Associations with histological features. Journal of Endocrinological Investigation. 2017;**40**(12):1327-1335. DOI: 10.1007/s40618-017-0700-4

[75] Al-Sharaky DR, Younes SF. Sensitivity and specificity of galectin-3 and glypican-3 in follicular-patterned and other thyroid neoplasms. Journal of Clinical and Diagnostic Research. 2016;**10**(3):EC06-EC10. DOI: 10.7860/JCDR/2016/18375.7430

[76] Zheng J, Lu W, Wang C, Xing Y, Chen X, Ai Z. Galectin-3 induced by hypoxia promotes cell migration in thyroid cancer cells. Oncotarget. 2017;**8**(60):101475-101488. DOI: 10.18632/oncotarget.21135

[77] Matesa-Anic D, Moslavac S, Matesa N, Cupic H, Kusic Z. Intensity and distribution of immunohistochemical expression of galectin-3 in thyroid neoplasms. Acta Clinica Croatica. 2012;**51**(2):237-241

[78] Arcolia V, Journe F, Wattier A, Leteurtre E, Renaud F, Gabius HJ, Remmelink M, Decaestecker C, Rodriguez A, Boutry S, Laurent S, Saussez S. Galectin-1 is a diagnostic marker involved in thyroid cancer progression. International Journal of Oncology. 2017;**51**(3):760-770. DOI: 10.3892/ijo.2017.4065

[79] Fanfone D, Despretz N, Stanicki D, Rubio-Magnieto J, Fossepre M, Surin M, Rorive S, Salmon I, Vander Elst L, Laurent S, Muller RN, Saussez S, Burtea C. Toward a new and noninvasive diagnostic method of papillary thyroid cancer by using peptide vectorised contrast agents targeted to galectin-1. Medical Oncology. 2017;**34**(11):184. DOI: 10.1007/s12032-017-1042-y

[80] Yamanaka K, Ito Y, Okuyama N, Noda K, Matsumoto H, Yoshida H, Miyauchi A, Capurro M, Filmus J, Miyoshi E. Immunohistochemical study of glypican 3 in thyroid cancer. Oncology. 2007;**73**(5-6):389-394. DOI: 10.1159/000136159

[81] Castellone MD, Celetti A, Guarino V, Cirafici AM, Basolo F, Giannini R, Medico E, Kruhoffer M, Orntoft TF, Curcio F, Fusco A, Melillo RM, Santoro M. Autocrine stimulation by osteopontin plays a pivotal role in the expression of the mitogenic and invasive phenotype of RET/PTC-transformed thyroid cells. Oncogene. 2004;**23**(12):2188-2196. DOI: 10.1038/sj.onc.1207322

[82] Guarino V, Faviana P, Salvatore G, Castellone MD, Cirafici AM, De Falco V, Celetti A, Giannini R, Basolo F, Melillo RM, Santoro M. Osteopontin is overexpressed in human papillary thyroid carcinomas and enhances thyroid carcinoma cell invasiveness. The Journal of Clinical Endocrinology and Metabolism. 2005;**90**(9):5270-5278. DOI: 10.1210/jc.2005-0271

[83] Wu G, Guo JJ, Ma ZY, Wang J, Zhou ZW, Wang Y. Correlation between calcification and bone sialoprotein and osteopontin in papillary thyroid carcinoma. International Journal of Clinical and Experimental Pathology. 2015;**8**(2):2010-2017

[84] Metivier KS, Deitz K, Xu WW, Conzemius M, Wilke VL. Gene expression profiling demonstrates differential expression of osteopontin in follicular thyroid carcinomas compared to normal thyroid tissue in dogs. Veterinary and Comparative Oncology. 2014;**12**(3):181-197. DOI: 10.1111/j.1476-5829.2012.00348.x

[85] Ferreira LB, Eloy C, Pestana A, Lyra J, Moura M, Prazeres H, Tavares C, Sobrinho-Simoes M, Gimba E, Soares P. Osteopontin expression is correlated with differentiation and good prognosis in medullary thyroid carcinoma. European Journal of Endocrinology. 2016;**174**(4):551-561. DOI: 10.1530/EJE-15-0577

[86] Wu G, Zhou Y, Li T, Guo J, Zhou Z. Immunohistochemical levels of matrix metalloproteinase-2 and CD44 variant 6 protein in the diagnosis and lateral cervical lymph node metastasis of papillary thyroid carcinoma. The Journal of International Medical Research. 2013;**41**(3):816-824. DOI: 10.1177/0300060513481923

[87] Calangiu CM, Simionescu CE, Stepan AE, Cernea D, Zavoi RE, Margaritescu C. The expression of CK19, vimentin and E-cadherin in differentiated thyroid carcinomas. Romanian Journal of Morphology and Embryology. 2014;**55**(3):919-925

[88] Ozolins A, Narbuts Z, Strumfa I, Volanska G, Stepanovs K, Gardovskis J. Immunohistochemical expression of HBME-1, E-cadherin, and CD56 in the differential diagnosis of thyroid nodules. Medicina (Kaunas, Lithuania). 2012;**48**(10):507-514

[89] Rendon-Huerta E, Chavarria-Velazquez CO, Montano LF. Claudins, inflammation and epithelial-mesenchymal transition in gastric tissue. Journal of Gastrointestinal and Digestive System. 2013;**3**:149. DOI: 10.4172/2161-069X.1000149

[90] Zwanziger D, Badziong J, Ting S, Moeller LC, Schmid KW, Siebolts U, Wickenhauser C, Dralle H, Fuehrer D. The impact of CLAUDIN-1 on follicular thyroid carcinoma aggressiveness. Endocrine-Related Cancer. 2015;**22**(5):819-830. DOI: 10.1530/ERC-14-0502

[91] Isic Dencic T, Cvejic D, Paunovic I, Tatic S, Havelka M, Savin S. Cytokeratin19 expression discriminates papillary thyroid carcinoma from other thyroid lesions and predicts its aggressive behaviour. Medical Oncology. 2013;**30**(1):362. DOI: 10.1007/s12032-012-0362-1

[92] Lamba Saini M, Bouzin C, Weynand B, Marbaix E. An appraisal of proliferation and apoptotic markers in papillary thyroid carcinoma: An automated analysis. PLoS One. 2016;**11**(2):e0148656. DOI: 10.1371/journal.pone.0148656

[93] Cyniak-Magierska A, Stasiak M, Naze M, Dedecjus M, Brzezinski J, Lewinski A. Patterns of cyclin A and B1 immunostaining in papillary thyroid carcinoma. Annals of Agricultural and Environmental Medicine. 2015;**22**(4):741-746. DOI: 10.5604/12321966.1185787

[94] Chen Z, Liu N, Zhu G, Dralle H, Hoang-Vu C. Targeting of the anti-apoptotic gene survivin in human thyroid carcinoma. International Journal of Molecular Medicine. 2012;**30**(3):465-472. DOI: 10.3892/ijmm.2012.1046

[95] Guerra A, Marotta V, Deandrea M, Motta M, Limone PP, Caleo A, Zeppa P, Esposito S, Fulciniti F, Vitale M. BRAF (V600E) associates with cytoplasmatic localization of p27kip1 and higher cytokeratin 19 expression in papillary thyroid carcinoma. Endocrine. 2013;**44**(1):165-171. DOI: 10.1007/s12020-012-9843-4

[96] Abulkheir IL, Mohammad DB. Value of immunohistochemical expression of p27 and galectin-3 in differentiation between follicular adenoma and follicular carcinoma. Applied Immunohistochemistry & Molecular Morphology. 2012;**20**(2):131-140. DOI: 10.1097/PAI.0b013e318228de00

[97] Pusztaszeri MP, Sadow PM, Faquin WC. CD117: A novel ancillary marker for papillary thyroid carcinoma in fine-needle aspiration biopsies. Cancer Cytopathology. 2014;**122**(8):596-603. DOI: 10.1002/cncy.21437

[98] Bychkov A, Jung CK. Aberrant expression of CD20 in thyroid cancer and its clinicopathologic significance. Human Pathology. 2018;**71**:74-83. DOI: 10.1016/j.humpath.2017.10.015

[99] Sasaki Y, Seto M, Miyoshi H, Okada S, Yokoyama S, Ohshima A, Ohshima K. Papillary thyroid carcinoma expressing CD20. Pathology International. 2017;**67**(7):350-354. DOI: 10.1111/pin.12548

[100] Wuertz FG, Kresnik E, Malle P, Hyden M, Lind P, Rogatsch H, Gallowitsch HJ. Fine-needle aspiration with immunohistochemistry using a modified scrape cell block technique for the diagnosis of thyroid and parathyroid nodules. Acta Cytologica. 2016;**60**(2):118-130. DOI: 10.1159/000446466

[101] Komminoth P, Roth J, Saremaslani P, Matias-Guiu X, Wolfe HJ, Heitz PU. Polysialic acid of the neural cell adhesion molecule in the human thyroid: A marker for medullary thyroid carcinoma and primary C-cell hyperplasia. An immunohistochemical study on 79 thyroid lesions. The American Journal of Surgical Pathology. 1994;**18**(4):399-411

[102] Frank-Raue K, Machens A, Leidig-Bruckner G, Rondot S, Haag C, Schulze E, Lorenz A, Kreissl MC, Dralle H, Raue F, Schmid KW. Prevalence and clinical spectrum of nonsecretory medullary thyroid carcinoma in a series of 839 patients with sporadic medullary thyroid carcinoma. Thyroid. 2013;**23**(3):294-300. DOI: 10.1089/thy.2012.0236

[103] Cappagli V, Potes CS, Ferreira LB, Tavares C, Eloy C, Elisei R, Sobrinho-Simoes M, Wookey PJ, Soares P. Calcitonin receptor expression in medullary thyroid carcinoma. PeerJ. 2017;**5**:e3778. DOI: 10.7717/peerj.3778

[104] Cvejic D, Savin S, Golubovic S, Paunovic I, Tatic S, Havelka M. Galectin-3 and carcinoembryonic antigen expression in medullary thyroid carcinoma: Possible relation to tumour progression. Histopathology. 2000;**37**(6):530-535

[105] Mourra N, Bennis M, Boelle PY, Cochand-Priollet B, Lefevre M, Lepine C, Balaton A, Klijanienko J, Menegaux F, Tissier F. Clusterin expression in medullary thyroid carcinoma is inversely correlated with the presence of lymph node metastases. Human Pathology. 2017;**64**:37-43. DOI: 10.1016/j.humpath.2017.03.009

[106] Werner TA, Tamkan-Olcek Y, Dizdar L, Riemer JC, Wolf A, Cupisti K, Verde PE, Knoefel WT, Krieg A. Survivin and XIAP: Two valuable biomarkers in medullary thyroid carcinoma. British Journal of Cancer. 2016;**114**(4):427-434. DOI: 10.1038/bjc.2016.5

[107] Lodewijk L, van Diest P, van der Groep P, Ter Hoeve N, Schepers A, Morreau J, Bonenkamp J, van Engen-van Grunsven A, Kruijff S, van Hemel B, Links T, Nieveen van Dijkum E, van Eeden S, Valk G, Borel Rinkes I, Vriens M. Expression of HIF-1α in medullary thyroid cancer identifies a subgroup with poor prognosis. Oncotarget. 2017;**8**(17):28650-28659. DOI: 10.18632/oncotarget.15622

[108] Bi Y, Meng Y, Wu H, Cui Q, Luo Y, Xue X. Expression of the potential cancer stem cell markers CD133 and CD44 in medullary thyroid carcinoma: A ten-year follow-up and

prognostic analysis. Journal of Surgical Oncology. 2016;**113**(2):144-151. DOI: 10.1002/jso.24124

[109] Herac M, Niederle B, Raderer M, Krebs M, Kaserer K, Koperek O. Expression of somatostatin receptor 2A in medullary thyroid carcinoma is associated with lymph node metastasis. Acta Pathologica, Microbiologica, et Immunologica Scandinavica. 2016;**124**(10):839-845. DOI: 10.1111/apm.12584

[110] Soudry E, Stern Shavit S, Hardy B, Morgenstern S, Hadar T, Feinmesser R. Heat shock proteins HSP90, HSP70 and GRP78 expression in medullary thyroid carcinoma. Annals of Diagnostic Pathology. 2017;**26**:52-56. DOI: 10.1016/j.anndiagpath.2016.11.003

[111] Melo DH, Mamede RCM, Neder L, Silva WA Jr, Barros-Filho MC, Kowalski LP, Pinto CAL, Zago MA, Figueiredo DLA, Jungbluth AA. Expression of cancer/testis antigens MAGE-A, MAGE-C1, GAGE and CTAG1B in benign and malignant thyroid diseses. Oncology Letters. 2017;**14**(6):6485-6496. DOI: 10.3892/ol.2017.7072

[112] Grimaldi A, Zarone MR, Irace C, Zappavigna S, Lombardi A, Kawasaki H, Caraglia M, Misso G. Non-coding RNAs as a new dawn in tumor diagnosis. Seminars in Cell & Developmental Biology. 2018;**78**:37-50. DOI: 10.1016/j.semcdb.2017.07.035

[113] MacFarlane LA, Murphy PR. MicroRNA: Biogenesis, function and role in cancer. Current Genomics. 2010;**11**(7):537-561. DOI: 10.2174/138920210793175895

[114] Hashemzadeh MR. Role of micro RNAs in stem cells, cardiac differentiation and cardiovascular diseases. Gene Reports. 2017;**8**:11-16

[115] Rodriguez-Montes JA, Menendez Sanchez P. Role of micro-RNA in colorectal cancer screening. Cirugía Española (English Edition). 2014;**92**(10):654-658. DOI: 10.1016/j.ciresp.2014.05.012

[116] Sasanakietkul T, Murtha TD, Javid M, Korah R, Carling T. Epigenetic modifications in poorly differentiated and anaplastic thyroid cancer. Molecular and Cellular Endocrinology. 2018;**469**:23-37. DOI: 10.1016/j.mce.2017.05.022

[117] Chruscik A, Lam AK. Clinical pathological impacts of microRNAs in papillary thyroid carcinoma: A crucial review. Experimental and Molecular Pathology. 2015;**99**(3):393-398. DOI: 10.1016/j.yexmp.2015.08.013

[118] Boufraqech M, Klubo-Gwiezdzinska J, Kebebew E. MicroRNAs in the thyroid. Best Practice & Research. Clinical Endocrinology & Metabolism. 2016;**30**(5):603-619. DOI: 10.1016/j.beem.2016.10.001

[119] Rossi ED, Martini M, Capodimonti S, Cenci T, Larocca LM. The role of miRNAs in the evaluation of follicular thyroid neoplasms: An overview of literature. Journal of the American Society of Cytopathology. 2017;**6**(3):96-104. DOI: https://doi.org/10.1016/j.jasc.2017.02.001

[120] Rodriguez-Rodero S, Delgado-Alvarez E, Diaz-Naya L, Martin Nieto A, Menendez Torre E. Epigenetic modulators of thyroid cancer. Endocrinology, Diabetes, Nutrition. 2017;**64**(1):44-56 . DOI: 10.1016/j.endinu.2016.09.006

[121] Hayashi M, Jono H, Shinriki S, Nakamura T, Guo J, Sueta A, Tomiguchi M, Fujiwara S, Yamamoto-Ibusuki M, Murakami K, Yamashita S, Yamamoto Y, Li JD, Iwase H, Ando Y. Clinical significance of CYLD downregulation in breast cancer. Breast Cancer Research and Treatment. 2014;**143**(3):447-457. DOI: 10.1007/s10549-013-2824-3

[122] Balkwill FR, Mantovani A. Cancer-related inflammation: Common themes and therapeutic opportunities. Seminars in Cancer Biology. 2012;**22**(1):33-40. DOI: 10.1016/j.semcancer.2011.12.005

[123] Strumfa I, Bogdanova T, Kalva A, Strumfs B, Rumba R, Vanags A, Drike I, Mezale D, Abolins A, Jakovlevs A, Balodis D, Gardovskis J. Systemic inflammatory reaction in gastric cancer: Biology and practical implications of neutrophil to lymphocyte ratio, Glasgow prognostic score and related parameters. In: Mozsik G, Karadi O, editors. Gastric Cancer. Croatia: InTech; 2017. pp. 143-197. DOI: 10.5772/intechopen.69723

[124] Roxburgh CS, McMillan DC. Role of systemic inflammatory response in predicting survival in patients with primary operable cancer. Future Oncology. 2010;**6**(1):149-163. DOI: 10.2217/fon.09.136

[125] McMillan DC. Systemic inflammation, nutritional status and survival in patients with cancer. Current Opinion in Clinical Nutrition and Metabolic Care. 2009;**12**(3):223-226. DOI: 10.1097/MCO.0b013e32832a7902

[126] Proctor MJ, Morrison DS, Talwar D, Balmer SM, Fletcher CD, O'Reilly DS, Foulis AK, Horgan PG, McMillan DC. A comparison of inflammation-based prognostic scores in patients with cancer. A Glasgow inflammation outcome study. European Journal of Cancer. 2011;**47**(17):2633-2641. DOI: 10.1016/j.ejca.2011.03.028

[127] Liu CL, Lee JJ, Liu TP, Chang YC, Hsu YC, Cheng SP. Blood neutrophil-to-lymphocyte ratio correlates with tumor size in patients with differentiated thyroid cancer. Journal of Surgical Oncology. 2013;**107**(5):493-497. DOI: 10.1002/jso.23270

[128] Kuo CY, Liu TP, Yang PS, Cheng SP. Characteristics of lymphocyte-infiltrating papillary thyroid cancer. Journal of Cancer Research and Practice. 2017;**4**(3):95-99